Robotic Surgery in Otolaryngology

Editors

NEIL D. GROSS
F. CHRIS HOLSINGER

OTOLARYNGOLOGIC CLINICS OF NORTH AMERICA

www.oto.theclinics.com

June 2014 • Volume 47 • Number 3

ELSEVIER

1600 John F. Kennedy Boulevard • Suite 1800 • Philadelphia, Pennsylvania, 19103-2899

http://www.oto.theclinics.com

OTOLARYNGOLOGIC CLINICS OF NORTH AMERICA Volume 47, Number 3
June 2014 ISSN 0030-6665, ISBN-13: 978-0-323-29927-5

Editor: Joanne Husovski
Developmental Editor: Susan Showalter

Otolaryngologic Clinics of North America (ISSN 0030-6665) is published bimonthly by Elsevier, Inc., 360 Park Avenue South, New York, NY 10010-1710. Months of issue are February, April, June, August, October, and December. Business and Editorial Offices: 1600 John F. Kennedy Blvd., Suite 1800, Philadelphia, PA 19103-2899. Customer Service Office: 6277 Sea Harbor Drive, Orlando, FL 32887-4800. Periodicals postage paid at New York, NY and additional mailing offices. Subscription prices is $365.00 per year (US individuals), $692.00 per year (US institutions), $175.00 per year (US student/resident), $485.00 per year (Canadian individuals), $876.00 per year (Canadian institutions), $540.00 per year (international individuals), $876.00 per year (international institutions), $270.00 per year (international & Canadian student/resident). Foreign air speed delivery is included in all *Clinics'* subscription prices. All prices are subject to change without notice. **POSTMASTER:** Send address changes to *Otolaryngologic Clinics of North America*, Elsevier Health Sciences Division, Subscription Customer Service, 3251 Riverport Lane, Maryland Heights, MO 63043. **Telephone: 1-800-654-2452 (U.S. and Canada); 314-447-8871 (outside U.S. and Canada). Fax: 314-447-8029. E-mail: journalscustomerservice-usa@elsevier.com (for print support); journalsonlinesupport-usa@elsevier.com (for online support).**

Reprints. For copies of 100 or more of articles in this publication, please contact the Commercial Reprints Department, Elsevier Inc., 360 Park Avenue South, New York, NY 10010-1710. Tel.: 212-633-3874; Fax: 212-633-3820; E-mail: reprints@elsevier.com.

Otolaryngologic Clinics of North America is also published in Spanish by McGraw-Hill Interamericana Editores S.A., P.O. Box 5-237, 06500 Mexico D.F., Mexico.

Otolaryngologic Clinics of North America is covered in *MEDLINE/PubMed (Index Medicus), Current Contents/Clinical Medicine, Excerpta Medica, BIOSIS, Science Citation Index,* and *ISI/BIOMED.*

Contributors

EDITORS

NEIL D. GROSS, MD, FACS
Associate Professor, Department of Otolaryngology-Head and Neck Surgery; Director of Head and Neck Robotic Surgery, Knight Cancer Institute, Oregon Health and Science University, Portland, Oregon

F. CHRISTOPHER HOLSINGER, MD, FACS
Professor and Chief, Division of Head and Neck Surgery; Professor, Department of Otolaryngology, Stanford University School of Medicine, Stanford Cancer Center, Palo Alto, California

AUTHORS

DANIEL BRICKMAN, MD
Fellow, Head and Neck Surgery, Department of Otolaryngology-Head and Neck Surgery, Oregon Health and Science University, Portland, Oregon

JASON Y.K. CHAN, MBBS
Resident, Department of Otolaryngology–Head and Neck Surgery, Johns Hopkins Hospital, Baltimore, Maryland

EUN CHANG CHOI, MD, PhD
Professor and Chairman, Department of Otorhinolaryngology, Yonsei University College of Medicine, Sedaemun-gu; Director, Yonsei Head and Neck Cancer Center, Severance Hospital, Yonsei University Health System, Seoul, South Korea

WOONG YOUN CHUNG, MD
Director of Minimally Invasive and Robotic Surgery, Severance Hospital; Associate Professor, Department of Surgery, Yonsei University School of Medicine, Seoul, Korea

JULIA A. CRAWFORD, MD
Head and Neck Surgery Center of Florida, Celebration Health, Florida Hospital, Celebration, Florida

NEIL D. GROSS, MD, FACS
Associate Professor, Department of Otolaryngology-Head and Neck Surgery; Director of Head and Neck Robotic Surgery, Knight Cancer Institute, Oregon Health and Science University, Portland, Oregon

EHAB HANNA, MD
Professor, Department of Head and Neck Surgery, MD Anderson Cancer Center, Houston, Texas

F. CHRISTOPHER HOLSINGER, MD, FACS
Professor and Chief, Division of Head and Neck Surgery; Professor, Department of Otolaryngology, Stanford University School of Medicine, Stanford Cancer Center, Palo Alto, California

YOON WOO KOH, MD, PhD
Associate Professor, Department of Otorhinolaryngology, Yonsei University College of Medicine, Sedaemun-gu, Seoul, South Korea

MICHAEL E. KUPFERMAN, MD
Associate Professor, Department of Head and Neck Surgery, MD Anderson Cancer Center, Houston, Texas

J. SCOTT MAGNUSON, MD
Head and Neck Surgery Center of Florida, Celebration Health, Florida Hospital, Celebration, Florida

FILIPPO MONTEVECHI, MD
Special Surgery Department, Otolaryngology-Head and Neck & Oral Surgery Unit, University of Pavia in Forlì, Morgagni Pierantoni Hospital, Forlì, Italy

JEREMY D. RICHMON, MD
Assistant Professor, Department of Otolaryngology–Head and Neck Surgery, Johns Hopkins Hospital, Baltimore, Maryland

MICHAEL C. SINGER, MD
Director, Division of Thyroid & Parathyroid Surgery, Department of Otolaryngology, Henry Ford Hospital, Detroit, Michigan

RICHARD V. SMITH, MD, FACS
Professor and Vice-Chair, Department of Otorhinolaryngology-Head and Neck Surgery; Director, Head and Neck Program, Montefiore Einstein Center for Cancer Care, Albert Einstein College of Medicine, Montefiore Medical Center, Bronx, New York

DAVID J. TERRIS, MD, FACS
Professor and Surgical Director of the GRU Thyroid Center, Department of Otolaryngology, Georgia Regents University, Augusta, Georgia

CLAUDIO VICINI, MD
Special Surgery Department, Otolaryngology-Head and Neck & Oral Surgery Unit, University of Pavia in Forlì, Morgagni Pierantoni Hospital, Forlì, Italy

Contents

 Videos of transoral robotic surgery (TORS) accompany this article

Treatment of squamous cell carcinoma of the oropharynx is challenging because of its effects on speech and swallowing, which may affect quality of life. Transoral robotic surgery may be an effective alternative to open surgery. Robotic lateral oropharyngectomy is best suited for early stage oropharyngeal squamous cell carcinoma, with the goal of avoiding or reducing the use or dose of adjuvant therapies. Successful robotic lateral oropharyngectomy requires appropriate training, detailed preoperative planning, organized operating room setup to obtain exposure, an understanding of the pertinent surgical anatomy, and knowledge of the postoperative care of the oncologic patient.

 A video of a surgeon confirming the dimensions of the working space before robotic thyroidectomy accompanies this article

Robotic thyroidectomy is ideal for patients with indeterminate, likely benign lesions less than 3 cm, and a body mass index less than 35 kg/mg^2. Proper arm position and padding are important to facilitate exposure and development of the working space from axilla to thyroid bed. The working space is developed using headlight and retractors without robotic assistance, establishing exposure of the thyroid bed from a 5-cm incision in the axilla. Three robotic instruments and a stereoscopic endoscope provide excellent visualization of the associated thyroid neurovasculature anatomy.

 Videos of a TORS supraglottic laryngectomy for a T2N0M0 squamous cell carcinoma using the Omniguide CO_2 laser and a TORS total laryngectomy accompany this article

Transoral robotic surgery (TORS) has become increasingly used to manage laryngeal and pharyngeal cancers, although the published experience in the larynx is small. Although there is burgeoning use of TORS for primary pharyngeal cancer, its application in the larynx is currently more limited. Successful TORS of the larynx has been predominantly as supraglottic laryngectomy, although there is some experience in total laryngectomy and cordectomy. Limitations of TORS of the larynx are primarily those of access and instrumentation, with respect to both the surgical robot and the retractors used to access the larynx transorally.

Nocturnal upper airway collapse is often multi-level in nature but typically will involve some degree of obstruction at the level of the tongue-base. Several surgical procedures have been developed in recent years to address this area in patients resistant to continuous positive airway pressure. This article outlines a novel way to treat obstructive sleep apnea lingual obstruction using the da Vinci robotic surgical system. This technique offers significant potential advantages over other established approaches and it should be included in the surgical armamentarium of sleep surgeons.

Transoral robotic surgery (TORS) offers a minimally invasive approach to the pharynx with a magnified 3-dimensional view, wristed instruments with 7 degrees of freedom, and tremor filtration. TORS affords an excellent approach to benign lesions of the pharynx. This article is grouped into subsites of the nasopharynx, oropharynx, and hypopharynx, addressing patient setup, surgical technique, and postoperative management of each subsite. Although TORS has been described primarily for resection of malignant lesions of the pharynx, the setup, exposure, and anatomy described herein are identical for benign lesions, the difference being the magnitude of resection.

Minimally invasive skull base surgery has advanced substantially with the advent of endoscopic technology, novel instrumentation, and intraoperative image-guidance capabilities. Robotic technology has been accepted into the surgeon's armamentarium, with its implementation into abdominal, thoracic, and head and neck surgery. However, the application of surgical robotics to the skull base has yet to be achieved. This article highlights current preclinical research and applications of robotic surgery to the skull base.

The use of minimally invasive and endoscopic thyroidectomy techniques has become widespread. However, these procedures all result in a visible neck incision. Several remote access thyroidectomy approaches that place the necessary incision in inconspicuous, noncervical locations have recently been described. Robotic facelift thyroidectomy uses a facelift incision in the postauricular area to provide entry to the thyroid compartment. Robotic facelift thyroidectomy has been shown to be feasible and safe and an increasing number of institutions have begun to offer it to selected patients. This article describes the indications, technical details, outcomes, and potential complications of this procedure.

Yoon Woo Koh and Eun Chang Choi

This article introduces and evaluates the feasibility of robot-assisted neck dissection as well as robot-assisted neck surgery via a modified facelift or retroauricular approach. Robot-assisted neck surgery is feasible compared with conventional techniques and shows a clear cosmetic benefit.

OTOLARYNGOLOGIC CLINICS
OF NORTH AMERICA

RELATED INTEREST

Oral and Maxillofacial Surgery Clinics, Volume 25, Issue 1, February 2013
Robotic Surgery: A New Approach to Tumors of the Tongue Base, Oropharynx, and Hypopharynx
John H. Campbell, *Editor*

DOWNLOAD
Free App!

Review Articles
THE CLINICS

NOW AVAILABLE FOR YOUR iPhone and iPad

Preface

Robotic Surgery of the Head and Neck

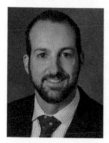 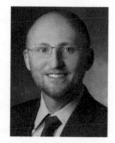

Neil D. Gross, MD   F. Chris Holsinger, MD
Editors

The role of robotics in surgery has yet to be defined. However, it is now evident that robotic technology has an established role for many procedures and will be increasingly important for less invasive and more precise delivery of surgical care in the future. For some surgical specialties, the incorporation of robotics has been dramatic. For example, most prostatectomies performed in the United States today are performed using robotic assistance.

This issue of *Otolaryngologic Clinics of North America* highlights the promise of robotic technology in otolaryngology. The role of robotics in otolaryngology has centered on transoral robotic surgery (TORS). The incorporation of TORS for benign and malignant neoplasms of the oropharynx has been palpable and is likely to expand, particularly for the treatment of obstructive sleep apnea. The role of robotics in otolaryngology beyond TORS remains uncertain.

The current platform for robotic surgery was not designed for use in otolaryngology. Therefore, there remain many challenges to implementing robotics in our specialty. For example, current technology lacks the haptic feedback critical for many procedures and is poorly suited for single-site access (eg, through the mouth). The current instruments are also useful only for soft tissue surgery, thereby excluding the majority of otologic and rhinologic procedures. Robotic technology will undoubtedly advance, hopefully spurred by increased competition in the marketplace and platforms specifically designed for otolaryngologic applications. In this manner, the current robotic platform can be viewed like the first generation of cell phones that were primitive compared with today's smartphones.

Regardless of technological advances, the rational incorporation of robotics in otolaryngology will require rigorous evaluation of outcomes and an honest appraisal by robotic surgeons in our specialty to define the potential added benefit of robotic assistance versus cost. Current NCI-funded clinical trials, RTOG 1221 and ECOG

Otolaryngol Clin N Am 47 (2014) ix–x
http://dx.doi.org/10.1016/j.otc.2014.03.005
0030-6665/14/$ – see front matter Published by Elsevier Inc.

oto.theclinics.com

3311, as well as smaller investigator-initiated outcome studies will play an important role in answering these questions. Thus, it is incumbent on leaders in robotic surgery in Otolaryngology to rise to this challenge by defining clear indications for robotic surgery as well as standardizing training and education for future robotic surgeons.

Neil D. Gross, MD
Head and Neck Surgery
Oregon Health and Science University
Portland, OR, USA

F. Chris Holsinger, MD
Head and Neck Surgery
Stanford University School of Medicine
Stanford, CA, US

E-mail addresses:
grossn@ohsu.edu (N.D. Gross)
holsinger@stanford.edu (F.C. Holsinger)

Robotic Approaches to the Pharynx: Tonsil Cancer

Daniel Brickman, MD, Neil D. Gross, MD*

KEYWORDS

- Robotic surgery • Transoral resection • Partial pharyngectomy • Tonsil cancer
- Squamous cell carcinoma

KEY POINTS

- Transoral robotic surgery (TORS) for tonsil cancer is an effective alternative to open surgery.
- Robotic lateral oropharyngectomy requires thorough understanding of oropharyngeal internal, parapharyngeal, and vascular anatomy.
- Preliminary reports have shown similar oncologic outcomes compared with historical surgical and nonsurgical treatments.
- The functional results of TORS compared with open surgical approaches show a decreased rate of permanent gastrostomy and tracheostomy tube dependence.

 Videos of transoral robotic surgery (TORS) accompany this article at http://www.oto.theclinics.com/

INTRODUCTION

It was estimated that 41,380 individuals (29,620 men and 11,760 women) would be diagnosed with and 7890 men and women would die of squamous cell carcinoma (SCC) of the oral cavity and pharynx in 2013.[1] Although the overall incidence of oral cavity and oropharynx SCC has been decreasing by approximately 1% per year, the incidence continues to increase in younger patients, because of the increasing incidence of human papillomavirus (HPV)-associated oropharyngeal SCC.[2] Treatment of oropharyngeal SCC is particularly challenging, because this site is involved in the crucial functions of breathing, deglutition, and speech. Impairment of any of these functions may significantly affect quality of life. Thus, both oncologic and functional outcomes are important considerations in the treatment of oropharyngeal SCC, including cancers that involve the tonsil.

Disclosures: None (D. Brickman); Intuitive Surgical, Proctor (N. Gross).
Department of Otolaryngology - Head and Neck Surgery, Oregon Health and Science University, Mail Code: PV01, 3181 Southwest Sam Jackson Park Road, Portland, OR 97239-3098, USA
* Corresponding author.
E-mail address: grossn@ohsu.edu

Otolaryngol Clin N Am 47 (2014) 359–372
http://dx.doi.org/10.1016/j.otc.2014.03.002
0030-6665/14/$ – see front matter Published by Elsevier Inc.
oto.theclinics.com

Traditional treatment of oropharyngeal cancers centered on surgical resection, which was often associated with significant morbidity. Several surgical options are available, with different exposures and associated morbidities. Mandibulotomy or mandibulectomy allow broad access to the oropharynx, but complication rates range from 10% to 60% and include difficulty with speech and swallowing, malocclusion, temporomandibular joint pain, and cosmetic deformity.[3-5] Lateral pharyngotomy, transhyoid pharyngotomy, or suprahyoid pharyngotomy may be used as an alternative to mandible splitting procedures. Patients undergoing pharyngotomy are at increased risk of pharyngocutaneous fistula formation and severe dysphagia, which has been reported to occur in 7% to 38% of patients.[6-8] Transoral resection provides the most direct route to the oropharynx, with the potential for decreased morbidity. The primary disadvantage of the transoral approach can be related to exposure, because of the need for direct line of sight. Many tonsil and pharyngeal cancers are difficult or impossible to reach through the mouth under direct vision. Acceptable oncologic outcomes have been reported using each of these approaches in selected patients (**Table 1**).[9]

Because of the difficult of exposure and potential for surgery-related morbidity, the treatment of oropharyngeal SCC in recent decades has evolved to a primary nonsurgical approach, namely chemoradiation. The Veterans Affairs study in 1991[10] heralded an era of organ preservation strategies, which have since been extrapolated from the larynx to the oropharynx. However, surgical approaches and techniques in head and neck cancer surgery have evolved dramatically. There is increased attention to functional preservation and use of minimally invasive procedures wherever feasible without compromising oncologic outcomes. Less radical procedures with minimal collateral tissue damage are preferred to decrease postoperative complications and to improve quality of life.

Several studies[11-14] have shown that transoral robotic surgery (TORS) may be an effective alternative to open surgery. The high-resolution, magnified, three-dimensional view of the operative field provided by TORS allows for excellent visualization of the target anatomy. TORS may overcome some limitations in exposure of surgical anatomy inherent in the direct line of site approach used in transoral laser microsurgery with its use of angled binocular endoscopic visualization. Additional advantages of TORS may include improved cosmesis, decreased length of hospital stay, and a low rate of gastrostomy tube dependence, improved long-term preservation of swallowing function, and ability to deintensify adjuvant therapy (**Table 2**).[15,16] High rates of negative surgical margins have been reported, which correlate well with local disease control (**Table 3**).[11,12,14]

TREATMENT GOALS

Current indications for robotic lateral oropharyngectomy include disease that is surgically resectable with negative margins. TORS is best suited for early stage SCC of the tonsil (T1-2, N0-1) with the goal of avoiding radiation therapy. In addition, advanced staged patients with low volume disease (T1-3, N1-2b) can be treated with the goal of avoiding adjuvant chemotherapy with planned postoperative radiation. Using these guidelines, the incidence of routine tracheotomy and prolonged gastrostomy tube use should be low.

PATIENT SELECTION

A thorough knowledge of the anatomy and appropriate robotic training are requisite to successful robotic lateral oropharyngectomy. Adequate exposure is also paramount. Before consideration of patients, potential deleterious patient factors must be

Table 1
Outcomes of traditional surgical approaches to the oropharynx

Study	Patients T Stage	Human Papillomavirus+	Tumor Site(s)	Primary Treatment Modality	Overall Survival (%)				Temporary/ Permanent Tracheostomy (%)	Temporary/ Permanent Gastrostomy Tube (%)
					1 y	1.5 y	2 y	>		
Sydney Head and Neck Cancer Institute[29]	92	NR	T1,2 OP	Surgery				83 (5 y)		
Hôpital de la Croix-Rousse[30]	53	NR	T1,2 OP	Surgery	100			73 (5 y)		
University of Paris[31,32]	191	NR	OP	Surgery	88			58 (5 y)	3.7/0	58.6/0
Mayo Clinic[33]	102	NR	OP	Surgery			92	85 (5 y)	34/4	14/1
University of Florida[34]	490	NR	OP	XRT				44 (5 y)		
MD Anderson Cancer Center[21]	150	NR	OP	XRT				47 (5 y)		
Total	1078				55				18/2	36/1

Abbreviations: NR, not reported; OP, oropharynx; XRT, radiotherapy.
Data from Refs.[21,29–34]

Table 2
Transoral robotic surgery functional outcomes

Study[a]	Patients	Tumor Site(s) T Stage	Temporary/ Permanent Tracheostomy (%)	Oral Diet Only Within 6 wk (%)	Temporary/ Permanent Gastrostomy Tube (%)	Preoperative/1 mo After MDADI	Baseline/3 mo/ 12 mo HNQOL
University of Pennsylvania[20]	47	OP T 1–4	11/0		0/2		
University of Alabama[11,13,21]	89	OC, OP, L T 1–4	3/0	79	25/0	77/61	
Mount Sinai Medical Center[12,22]	30	OP, L T 1–2	13/0				76.3/61.2/76.8
Mayo Clinic[14,23,24]	66	OP T 1–3	26/2	97	27/5		
Ohio State University[25–27]	81	OP T 1–3		100	21/9		78.7/67.9/77.9
Total	313		13/1	92	18/4		

Abbreviations: HNQOL, Head and Neck Quality of Life instrument; L, larynx; MDADI, MD Anderson Dysphagia Inventory; OC, oral cavity; OP, oropharynx.
[a] Consecutive institutional studies summarized. Maximum number of study patients cited.
Data from Refs.[11–14,20–27]

Table 3
Transoral robotic surgery oncologic outcomes

Study	Patients T Stage	Human Papillomavirus +	Overall Survival (%)				Disease-Specific Survival (%)				Recurrence-Free Survival (%)			
			1 y	1.5 y	2 y	>	1 y	1.5 y	2 y	>	1 y	1.5 y	2 y	>
University of Alabama[21]	89 T 1–4										89	86		92 (3 y)
University of Pennsylvania[28]	50 T 1–4	74	96		81		98		93					
Mount Sinai Medical Center[22]	30 T 1–2			90								78		
Ohio State University[23]	66 T 1–3	67				96 (3 y)				95 (3 y)				
Mayo Clinic[25]	81 T 1–3	72							92	89 (4 y)				
Total	316	71												

Data from Refs.[21–23,25,28]

considered, including obstructive dentition, trismus, and kyphosis. For these reasons, some experienced TORS surgeons recommend routine staging endoscopy. This added surgical step may be unnecessary with experience. Likewise, some surgeons prefer to stage the neck dissection several weeks before or after a TORS resection for tonsillar cancer to avoid the risk of intraoperative pharyngocutaneous fistula. A staged procedure is appropriate if level 1b is planned for dissection. Otherwise, the neck dissection can be performed safely at the time of resection of the primary. Even if a fistula is created during TORS, immediate surgical repairs are highly successful.

The major tumor-related contraindications include mandibular invasion, tongue base involvement requiring resection of greater than 50% of the tongue base, and pharyngeal wall involvement necessitating resection of more than 50% of the posterior pharyngeal wall in addition to typical definitions of unresectabililty (carotid encasement, skull base/brain invasion, spine invasion).[17] Relative contraindications to upfront surgical treatment with robotic resection of tonsillar cancer may also include cervical lymphadenopathy, with gross extracapsular extension on preoperative imaging and large primary tumor size or extent precluding the realistic possibility of negative surgical margins.

PREOPERATIVE PLANNING AND SPECIAL EQUIPMENT

Preoperative cross-sectional imaging is imperative. Computed tomography (CT) scans can help identify a medially placed carotid system (**Fig. 1**), gross tumor involvement of the carotid, prevertebral involvement, and burden of cervical disease. A CT angiogram may be helpful for delineating the complex vascular anatomy of the oropharynx and parapharyngeal space. Positron emission tomography can also be useful for identification of pathologic retropharyngeal lymph nodes or contralateral cervical adenopathy.

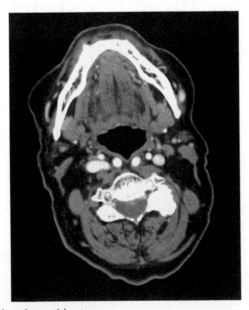

Fig. 1. Medially displaced carotid artery.

Proper patient positioning and setup is critical for a successful robotic operation. The operating table is reversed and capable of being turned 180° to allow the robot support legs to fit under the bed. Intubation can be transnasal or transoral. A shoulder roll can help with exposure, although contralateral nasal intubation is preferred. Arm tucking and draping are optional. A large silk suture placed across the anterior tongue can be used to manipulate the tongue during suspension laryngoscopy to maximize exposure. Standard retractors (eg, Crow-Davis, Dingman) provide adequate exposure for most cancers limited to the tonsil. The Feyh-Kastenbauer laryngeal retractor (Gyrus AMI, Southborough, MA), allows for superior visualization at the inferior extent of disease, which often includes the glossotonsillar fold and lateral base of tongue. The retractor can be stabilized using any available suspension device, including dedicated laryngoscope holders. A red rubber catheter can be placed through the contralateral nare to provide traction on the soft palate.

Careful positioning of the robotic patient cart is important to maximize instrument degree of freedom and minimize robotic arm collisions. The bed must be lowered to accommodate the robotic arms over the suspension apparatus. The da Vinci S or Si Surgical System (Intuitive Surgical, Sunnyvale, CA) patient cart with robotic arms is positioned under the head of the bed with approximately 30° of rotation. Robotic lateral oropharyngectomy uses only 3 of the 4 interactive robotic arms: 1 camera (central), 2 working instruments (lateral). Zero-degree and 30-degree cameras are available, but the 0-degree is most useful for tonsil cases for better visualization of the superior pole. The 30-degree camera can be used to improve exposure of the glossotonsillar fold and base of tongue. Monopolar cautery is placed ipsilateral to the tumor and a Maryland dissecting forceps (Intuitive Surgical, Sunnyvale, CA) in the working arm contralateral to the tumor to provide traction. The instrument arms are placed in a V formation surrounding the central camera (**Fig. 2**).

A properly trained surgical assistant in addition to the scrub nurse is important during TORS. The assistant must have endoscopic skills because they are working from a screen rather than direct visualization. Further, the assistant must be familiar enough with the robotic instruments to help troubleshoot potential device malfunction or robotic arm interference. The assistant can be equipped with suction Bovie, laryngeal suction, and an endoscopic clip applier (eg, 22-cm Karl Storz Steiner clip forceps, Tuttlingen, Germany). The primary role of the assistant is to suction smoke and blood. The assistant is also critical for clipping vessels, retracting, and applying external hyoid pressure intermittently, as directed by the primary surgeon.

PROCEDURE

The procedure is started with direct laryngoscopy with or without esophagoscopy, unless a staging endoscopy has been already performed. The patient is positioned and suspension laryngoscopy is performed. The robotic patient cart, surgical arms, and assistant are positioned. Before incision, the camera and robotic arms should be maneuvered to check for responsiveness and adequate degrees of freedom.

The initial mucosal cut is made starting at the palate or superior pole of the tonsil and extended from superior to inferior along the lateral aspect of the anterior tonsillar pillar and pterygomandibular raphe (**Fig. 3**, Video 1). As with open procedures, a 1-cm margin of normal-appearing mucosa is included in the resection. Dissection is then carried through the submucosal muscle layers, palatoglossus and palatopharyngeus muscles superiorly, and superior constrictor muscle anterolaterally. Adequate traction and countertraction can be achieved with the assistance of a nasal red rubber catheter or intermittent lateral retraction by the surgical assistant using a

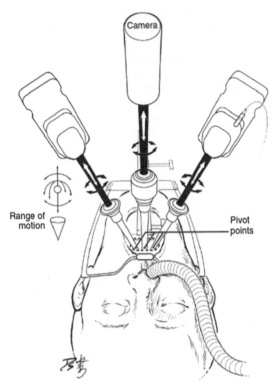

Fig. 2. Positioning of the robotic arms. (*From* Gross ND, Holsinger FC, Magnuson JS, et al. Transoral robotic surgery. In: Cohen JI, Clayman GL, editors. Atlas of head and neck surgery. New York: Elsevier; 2011. p. 300; with permission.)

Hurd tonsil dissector/pillar retractor. At this point, the Maryland dissector can be used to bluntly push the specimen and avoid tearing the mucosa and muscle overlying the tumor edges.

Blunt dissection is used to traverse the buccopharyngeal fascia and enter the parapharyngeal space laterally (**Fig. 4**, Video 2). The parapharyngeal space is identified by the presence of parapharyngeal fat. The medial pterygoid muscle may be visualized first and found immediately cephalad to the parapharyngeal fat. Identification of this structure allows the surgeon to assess the superolateral extent of disease. It is usually possible to visualize carotid pulsations at this point deep and lateral to the parapharyngeal fat. Further dissection laterally should be avoided to minimize exposure of the carotid artery.

At this point, numerous branches of the external carotid system that traverse the parapharyngeal space to enter the constrictor muscles are encountered (**Fig. 5**, Video 3). Any vessel larger than 1 mm is meticulously clipped and divided to minimize the risk of postoperative bleeding. The tonsillar branch of the lesser palatine artery and vein is usually encountered first superiorly and can be variable in size. The tonsillar branches of the ascending pharyngeal and ascending palatine arteries can be visualized more inferiorly.

Dissection is continued from superior to inferior using cautery to divide the remaining superior pharyngeal constrictor muscle. The buccopharyngeal fascia is left intact laterally when possible. Increased caution in this area is advised to avoid the carotid,

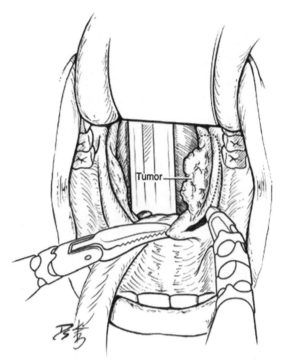

Fig. 3. Initial mucosal cut. (*From* Gross ND, Holsinger FC, Magnuson JS, et al. Transoral robotic surgery. In: Cohen JI, Clayman GL, editors. Atlas of head and neck surgery. New York: Elsevier; 2011. p. 301; with permission.)

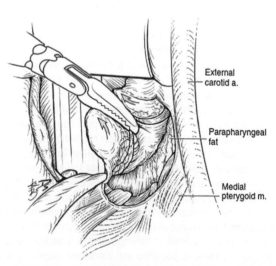

Fig. 4. Identification of the parapharyngeal space. a, artery; m, muscle. (*From* Gross ND, Holsinger FC, Magnuson JS, et al. Transoral robotic surgery. In: Cohen JI, Clayman GL, editors. Atlas of head and neck surgery. New York: Elsevier; 2011. p. 303; with permission.)

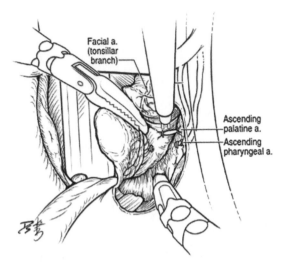

Fig. 5. Apply vascular clips. a, artery. (*From* Gross ND, Holsinger FC, Magnuson JS, et al. Transoral robotic surgery. In: Cohen JI, Clayman GL, editors. Atlas of head and neck surgery. New York: Elsevier; 2011. p. 303; with permission.)

which can be found more medial at the inferior limits of the dissection. The tonsillar branch of the facial artery is traversed at the inferior portion of the dissection.

The inferior mucosal cuts are made after judging the extent of disease. The dissection may include the glossotonsillar fold and base of tongue, depending on the extent of disease. In addition, a 30-degree scope facing the base of tongue can improve exposure. Assistant retraction or external hyoid pressure may also be necessary at this point to fully visualize the tumor. Rarely, adjustment or repositioning of the laryngoscope with possible removal and replacement of the robotic arms may be needed to ensure adequate exposure for surgical margins.

Rolling the specimen from lateral to medial, the pharyngeal constrictor muscle, styloglossus, and glossopharyngeus muscles can be divided from superior to inferior (**Fig. 6**, Video 4). A branch of the glossopharyngeal nerve can be identified between the muscle layers, which can be preserved in many cases. Occasionally, a tonsillar branch of the dorsal lingual artery can be encountered as well, further highlighting the vascular complexity and variability of the area. The final mucosal cuts are then completed medially along the posterior pharyngeal wall to ensure adequate radial margins. The specimen is dissected off the prevertebral fascia again from lateral to medial, and the constrictor muscles are divided along the medial attachment.

The specimen can then be removed. An en bloc resection is feasible in most cases. However, bulky tumors that traverse the glossotonsillar fold may be better extirpated in 2 pieces. It is important to maintain orientation of the specimen to allow accurate pathologic assessment. Some investigators advocate inking resection margins in the operating room. Others routinely send frozen sections for margin analysis, especially in large tumors, or send separate margins for permanent section analyses.

The wound is inspected for hemostasis before removing the robotic instruments and taking the patient out of suspension laryngoscopy. The liberal use of further clips, unipolar, or bipolar cautery here is paramount, because bleeding after TORS can be life threatening. Many surgeons routinely place a nasogastric feeding tube at the conclusion of the procedure. For others, the need for postoperative feeding assistance is dictated by the extent of resection, comorbidities, and nutritional status.

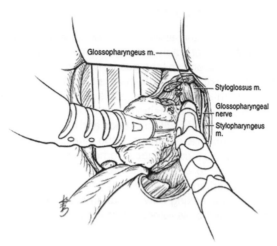

Fig. 6. Divide deep pharyngeal muscles as needed. m, muscle. (*From* Gross ND, Holsinger FC, Magnuson JS, et al. Transoral robotic surgery. In: Cohen JI, Clayman GL, editors. Atlas of head and neck surgery. New York: Elsevier; 2011. p. 304; with permission.)

Neck dissection is routinely offered. It can be performed at the same time as the TORS portion of the procedure, with little morbidity.[18] Some surgeons prefer to stage the neck dissection before or after TORS to avoid creating a connection between the pharynx and neck as well as to avoid additional laryngopharyngeal swelling, which might result in the need for a tracheotomy.

COMPLICATIONS

Early reports of TORS oropharyngeal resections reported complication rates as high as 19%.[17] In the largest series of TORS to date,[19] no mortalities were reported. A wide range of concomitant tracheotomy during TORS resection has been reported, with incidences from 0% to 31%.[12,14] Unplanned tracheostomy and reintubations have also been reported in up to 3.7%.[17] The most dangerous major complication is bleeding from the primary site. It can present as minor mucosal edge bleeding, which is easily controlled with suction Bovie, to major arterial bleeding from the external carotid system. Reported bleeding incidence rates range from 0% to 7.5%.[4,16] Minor complications after resection of the primary include the development of nasal regurgitation with hypernasality, lingual nerve numbness, postoperative trismus, and cervicalgia.[17] All patients experience significant temporary dysphagia and odynophagia.

In addition to standard risks of neck dissection, primary resection in the oropharynx yields the risk for pharyngeal communication with the neck, with possible pharyngo-cutaneous fistula formation. One study of 148 patients[18] noted a 29% chance of oro-cervical communication intraoperatively when the robotic resected tonsillar primary tumors and unilateral tongue base tumors were coupled with ipsilateral level I to IV neck dissections. All were managed with some combination of primary closure, local tissue advancement, fibrin glue application, and cervical drain placement. Of these patients, 6 (4%) developed a subcutaneous pharyngeal fluid accumulation requiring postoperative management via controlled incision and drainage with daily packing placement. No patients experienced a delay in adjuvant therapy and had similar cosmetic outcomes per the investigators.

POSTPROCEDURAL CARE AND RECOVERY

At completion of the procedure, the airway should be carefully evaluated, with consideration of overnight intubation or tracheostomy as needed. Long surgical times and tongue compression from suspension laryngoscopy have been known to cause significant tongue edema. Once extubated, patients are monitored in the hospital until sufficient pain control and nutritional support is achieved, typically more than 48 hours.

If a feeding tube was placed, the position should be confirmed by imaging before use. After surgery, the patient works with a speech and language pathologist to assess swallowing safety and promote rehabilitation. If the patient tolerates a diet sufficient to support their caloric needs, the feeding tube is removed in the hospital. All patients are seen in clinic within 1 week to check their progress and remove feeding tubes if needed. Drains are managed and removed with similar criteria to other neck procedures, with care to note that leaking may signal an orocervical fistula. Perioperative steroids may be useful to decrease expected oropharyngeal edema and postoperative nausea and vomiting.

OUTCOMES

Robotic lateral oropharyngectomy, including selective neck dissection, provides the most accurate staging information for tonsillar SCC. Improved risk stratification with pathologic staging may allow for deintensification of adjuvant therapies.[15] In particular, a reduction in postoperative radiation dose to 54 to 60 Gy, rather than a definitive treatment dose of 66 to 70 Gy, is believed to reduce the potential for long-term toxicities. Although long-term outcomes data are lacking, there is evidence showing a direct correlation between radiation dose and apical peridontitis.[15] In addition, a survival benefit has been associated with surgical treatment before radiation therapy in early stage tonsil SCC.[35] Further rigorous studies are still required to validate these innovative approaches and to define their optimal usefulness in patients with tonsillar SCC and other malignancies of the oropharynx.

Compared with historic surgical and nonsurgical controls, robotic lateral oropharyngectomy seems to have comparable rates of disease control (**Tables 1–3**). These comparisons are confounded by their lack of information regarding HPV status and selection bias in staging of patients chosen for surgery. Overall survival varies widely in terms of presenting stage: from 89% for stage I tumors to 52% for stage IV.[36] Overall, improved functional results in terms of long-term dependence on gastrostomy and tracheostomy tubes have been shown in TORS patients compared with their open approach counterparts.

SUMMARY

Management of tonsillar SCC remains challenging in part because of multiple treatment options and the evolution of technology, including TORS. Given the expected excellent oncologic outcome of most patients with tonsil cancer, minimizing treatment morbidity is a significant consideration in assessing new treatment modalities for tonsillar SCC. Surgical innovations, including TORS, offer the potential for improved preservation of speech and swallowing without compromising survival. Recent literature supports the feasibility of TORS for surgical resection of tonsillar SCC. Using robotic lateral oropharyngectomy, appropriately selected cancers involving the tonsil can be safely resected with negative margins, without the use of routine tracheotomy, and without a high risk of permanent gastrostomy tube need.

SUPPLEMENTARY DATA

Supplementary data related to this article can be found online at http://dx.doi.org/10.1016/j.otc.2014.03.002.

REFERENCES

1. Howlader N. Noone AM. Krapcho M. et al. SEER cancer statistics review, 1975-2010. Bethesda (MD): National Cancer Institute. Accessed November 13, 2013.
2. Brown LM, Check DP, Devesa SS. Oral cavity and pharynx cancer incidence trends by subsite in the United States: changing gender patterns. J Oncol 2012;2012:649498.
3. Dziegielewski PT, Mlynarek AM, Dimitry J, et al. The mandibulotomy: friend or foe? Safety outcomes and literature review. Laryngoscope 2009;119(12): 2369-75.
4. Babin R, Calcaterra TC. The lip-splitting approach to resection of oropharyngeal cancer. J Surg Oncol 1976;8(5):433-6.
5. Sessions DG. Surgical resection and reconstruction for cancer of the base of the tongue. Otolaryngol Clin North Am 1983;16(2):309-29.
6. Nasri S, Oh Y, Calcaterra TC. Transpharyngeal approach to base of tongue tumors: a comparative study. Laryngoscope 1996;106(8):945-50.
7. Moore DM, Calcaterra TC. Cancer of the tongue base treated by a transpharyngeal approach. Ann Otol Rhinol Laryngol 1990;99(4 Pt 1):300-3.
8. Zeitels SM, Vaughan CW, Ruh S. Suprahyoid pharyngotomy for oropharynx cancer including the tongue base. Arch Otolaryngol Head Neck Surg 1991;117(7): 757-60.
9. Laccourreye O, Benito J, Garcia D, et al. Lateral pharyngotomy for selected cancer of the lateral oropharynx. Part II: when and why. Laryngoscope 2013;123(11): 2718-22.
10. Induction chemotherapy plus radiation compared with surgery plus radiation in patients with advanced laryngeal cancer. The Department of Veterans Affairs Laryngeal Cancer Study Group. N Engl J Med 1991;324(24):1685-90.
11. Boudreaux BA, Rosenthal EL, Magnuson JS, et al. Robot-assisted surgery for upper aerodigestive tract neoplasms. Arch Otolaryngol Head Neck Surg 2009; 135(4):397-401.
12. Genden EM, Desai S, Sung CK. Transoral robotic surgery for the management of head and neck cancer: a preliminary experience. Head Neck 2009;31(3):283-9.
13. Iseli TA, Kulbersh BD, Iseli CE, et al. Functional outcomes after transoral robotic surgery for head and neck cancer. Otolaryngol Head Neck Surg 2009;141(2): 166-71.
14. Moore EJ, Olsen KD, Kasperbauer JL. Transoral robotic surgery for oropharyngeal squamous cell carcinoma: a prospective study of feasibility and functional outcomes. Laryngoscope 2009;119(11):2156-64.
15. Weinstein GS, Quon H, O'Malley BW Jr, et al. Selective neck dissection and deintensified postoperative radiation and chemotherapy for oropharyngeal cancer: a subset analysis of the University of Pennsylvania transoral robotic surgery trial. Laryngoscope 2010;120(9):1749-55.
16. Weinstein GS, O'Malley BW Jr, Magnuson JS, et al. Transoral robotic surgery: a multicenter study to assess feasibility, safety, and surgical margins. Laryngoscope 2012;122(8):1701-7.
17. Weinstein GS, O'Malley BW Jr, Snyder W, et al. Transoral robotic surgery: radical tonsillectomy. Arch Otolaryngol Head Neck Surg 2007;133(12):1220-6.

18. Moore EJ, Olsen KD, Martin EJ. Concurrent neck dissection and transoral robotic surgery. Laryngoscope 2011;121(3):541–4.
19. Asher SA, White HN, Kejner AE, et al. Hemorrhage after transoral robotic-assisted surgery. Otolaryngol Head Neck Surg 2013;149(1):112–7.
20. Weinstein GS, O'Malley BW Jr, Cohen MA, et al. Transoral robotic surgery for advanced oropharyngeal carcinoma. Arch Otolaryngol Head Neck Surg 2010; 136(11):1079–85.
21. White HN, Moore EJ, Rosenthal EL, et al. Transoral robotic-assisted surgery for head and neck squamous cell carcinoma: one- and 2-year survival analysis. Arch Otolaryngol Head Neck Surg 2010;136(12):1248–52.
22. Genden EM, Kotz T, Tong CC, et al. Transoral robotic resection and reconstruction for head and neck cancer. Laryngoscope 2011;121(8):1668–74.
23. Moore EJ, Olsen SM, Laborde RR, et al. Long-term functional and oncologic results of transoral robotic surgery for oropharyngeal squamous cell carcinoma. Mayo Clin Proc 2012;87(3):219–25.
24. Olsen SM, Moore EJ, Laborde RR, et al. Transoral surgery alone for human-papillomavirus-associated oropharyngeal squamous cell carcinoma. Ear Nose Throat J 2013;92(2):76–83.
25. Dziegielewski PT, Teknos TN, Durmus K, et al. Transoral robotic surgery for oropharyngeal cancer: long-term quality of life and functional outcomes. JAMA Otolaryngol Head Neck Surg 2013;139:1–9.
26. Hurtuk A, Agrawal A, Old M, et al. Outcomes of transoral robotic surgery: a preliminary clinical experience. Otolaryngol Head Neck Surg 2011;145(2):248–53.
27. Hurtuk AM, Marcinow A, Agrawal A, et al. Quality-of-life outcomes in transoral robotic surgery. Otolaryngol Head Neck Surg 2012;146(1):68–73.
28. Cohen MA, Weinstein GS, O'Malley BW Jr, et al. Transoral robotic surgery and human papillomavirus status: oncologic results. Head Neck 2011;33(4):573–80.
29. Moncrieff M, Sandilla J, Clark J, et al. Outcomes of primary surgical treatment of T1 and T2 carcinomas of the oropharynx. Laryngoscope 2009;119(2):307–11.
30. Cosmidis A, Rame JP, Dassonville O, et al. T1-T2 N0 oropharyngeal cancers treated with surgery alone. A GETTEC study. Eur Arch Otorhinolaryngol 2004; 261(5):276–81.
31. Laccourreye O, Hans S, Menard M, et al. Transoral lateral oropharyngectomy for squamous cell carcinoma of the tonsillar region: II. An analysis of the incidence, related variables, and consequences of local recurrence. Arch Otolaryngol Head Neck Surg 2005;131(7):592–9.
32. Holsinger FC, McWhorter AJ, Menard M, et al. Transoral lateral oropharyngectomy for squamous cell carcinoma of the tonsillar region: I. Technique, complications, and functional results. Arch Otolaryngol Head Neck Surg 2005;131(7): 583–91.
33. Moore EJ, Henstrom DK, Olsen KD, et al. Transoral resection of tonsillar squamous cell carcinoma. Laryngoscope 2009;119(3):508–15.
34. Fein DA, Lee WR, Amos WR, et al. Oropharyngeal carcinoma treated with radiotherapy: a 30-year experience. Int J Radiat Oncol Biol Phys 1996;34(2):289–96.
35. Holliday MA, Tavaluc R, Zhuang T, et al. Oncologic benefit of tonsillectomy in stage I and II tonsil cancer: a surveillance epidemiology and end results database review. JAMA Otolaryngol Head Neck Surg 2013;139(4):362–6.
36. Galati LT, Myers EN, Johnson JT. Primary surgery as treatment for early squamous cell carcinoma of the tonsil. Head Neck 2000;22(3):294–6.

Robotic Thyroidectomy

F. Christopher Holsinger, MD[a],*, Woong Youn Chung, MD[b]

KEYWORDS

- Robotic • Thyroidectomy • Transaxillary

KEY POINTS

- Robotic thyroidectomy is ideal for patients with indeterminate, likely benign lesions less than 3 cm, and a body mass index less than 35 kg/mg^2.
- Informed consent should include a clarification that robotic thyroidectomy is currently considered an off-label use of the da Vinci Surgical System in the United States.
- Careful attention to arm position and proper padding before the procedure is important to facilitate exposure and development of the working space from axilla to thyroid bed.
- The working space is developed using headlight and retractors without robotic assistance, establishing exposure of the thyroid bed from a 5-cm incision in the axilla.
- Three robotic instruments and a stereoscopic endoscope provide excellent visualization of the associated thyroid neurovasculature anatomy.

 A video of a surgeon confirming the dimensions of the working space before robotic thyroidectomy accompanies this article at http://www.oto.theclinics.com/

INDICATIONS

Patients with an indication for unilateral thyroid lobectomy may be candidates for robotic thyroidectomy. Surgeons considering this approach should have extensive experience in head and neck endocrine surgery, and familiarity with the lateral neck and pectoralis major muscle. Contraindications include tumors greater than 3 to 5 cm and/or lesions located more deeply and posteriorly in the tracheoesophageal groove. The patient's body habitus and body mass index (BMI) are also important considerations, because the transaxillary approach in patients with a low BMI (<35 kg/mg^2) is much easier and faster to perform. If the distance between the axillary incision and thyroid is greater than 18 to 20 cm, establishing and maintaining an adequate working space may be difficult. In addition, coexisting Hashimoto thyroiditis and Graves disease may also be relative contraindications. Great caution should be taken when using the transaxillary approach for lesions that extend to the posterior aspect of the thyroid adjacent to the tracheoesophageal groove, because an increased risk may be present

[a] Division of Head and Neck Surgery, Stanford University School of Medicine, 875 Blake Wilbur Drive, CC-2227, Palo Alto, CA 94304-2205, USA; [b] Department of Surgery, Severance Hospital, Yonsei University School of Medicine, 50-1 Yonsei-Ro SeoDaemun-Gu, Seoul 120-752, Korea
* Corresponding author.
E-mail address: holsinger@ohns.stanford.edu

Otolaryngol Clin N Am 47 (2014) 373–378
http://dx.doi.org/10.1016/j.otc.2014.03.001
0030-6665/14/$ – see front matter © 2014 Elsevier Inc. All rights reserved.

oto.theclinics.com

for injury to the trachea, esophagus, and recurrent laryngeal nerve. The role of robotic thyroidectomy for malignancy is currently not well studied in the United States.

Surgeons should thoroughly discuss the risks and benefits of robotic thyroidectomy, presenting a balanced approach to the patient. Informed consent should include a clarification that robotic thyroidectomy is currently considered an off-label use of the da Vinci Surgical System in the United States.

SURGICAL TECHNIQUE
Axillary Incision and Approach

While the patient is sitting in an upright position, just before surgery, the incision should be outlined in the holding area to best camouflage the scar.

- First, the inferior limit of the incision is identified by a horizontal line drawn from the sternal notch laterally to the folds of the axilla. Chung recommends then drawing an oblique line 60° from the midline from just above the laryngeal prominence of the thyroid cartilage and thyrohyoid membrane to the axilla.
- Depending on patient-specific anatomic landmarks within the axilla and body habitus, a gentle taper or even a C-shaped incision can be considered to accommodate the incision into the relaxed skin tension lines of the axilla.

Surgical Note: Close coordination with the anesthesia team is important for laryngeal nerve monitoring and to optimize patient arm and shoulder positioning.

- For robotic thyroidectomy, the authors prefer to use an endotracheal tube with a laryngeal nerve monitor.
- After general anesthesia is induced with the patient in supine position, the authors confirm that the incision is hidden well by placing the arm in a comfortable resting position, as initially described by Chung.
- The ipsilateral arm is then gently rotated nearly 180° cephalad, placed on an armboard, and carefully padded.

Surgical Note: Great care must be taken to minimize stretch injury of the brachial plexus from hyperextending the arm or overly rotating the arm medially. Ikeda and colleagues described a comfortable position for the arm to minimize these complications.

- Whether using Chung's (**Fig. 1**A) or Ikeda's approach (see **Fig. 1**B), proper patient positioning rotates the clavicle superiorly, effectively reducing the distance between the axilla and the thyroid.
- Padding the forearm and especially the elbow is essential to prevent neuropraxia and stretch injury.
- The arm and shoulder should be at the same vertical height, further minimizing risk for neuropraxia.
- Finally, the use of a thyroid pillow may be optimal for providing neuromuscular support, because this platform supports not only the neck and shoulder but also the scapula and upper back.
- Covered with sterile drapes, the da Vinci patient cart is positioned on the contralateral side of the operating table.
- The arm is secured with tape, and the neck, axilla, and upper chest are prepared and draped in standard sterile fashion.
- A 5-cm skin incision is made in the axilla just lateral to the anterior transaxillary fold at the posterior border of the pectoralis major muscle, as outlined earlier, both parallel to but lateral to the lateral edge of the pectoralis major muscle.

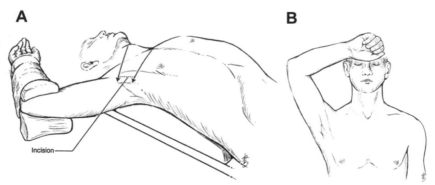

Fig. 1. (*A*) The position for robotic thyroidectomy described by Chung, with the arm turned and straight, carefully supported with padding at the patient's side. (*B*) The position for endoscopic thyroidectomy described by Ikeda and colleagues, with the arm curved and resting over the patient's head or at the head of the operating room table. The *arrows* outline the extent of the working space required to gain adequate exposure. (*From* Holsinger FC, Zafereo ME, Chung WY. Robotic thyroidectomy: surgical technique for lobectomy via axillary incision without carbon dioxide insufflation. In: Cohen JI, Clayman GL, editors. Atlas of head and neck surgery. New York: Elsevier; 2011. p. 491; with permission.)

- The authors then establish a working space in a subcutaneous plane, superficial to the pectoralis major muscle fascia toward the clavicle.

Surgical Note: It is important to stay superficial to this fascia of the pectoralis major muscle at all times to minimize muscle fiber injury and postoperative seroma. Across the bed, the surgical assistant uses a series of retractors, ranging from Army-Navy to the Sauerbruch, and even extended-length Devers, which are required to develop the working space from axilla to thyroid bed.

- An extended needle-tip electrocautery handpiece is required as the working space is established medially.
- The authors use 1 or 2 lighted breast retractors with inline suction to evacuate smoke and thus improve exposure; a headlight can also improve visualization. This stage is when patients with high BMI present several challenges for the surgeon in establishing the working space.

Surgical Note: During the establishment of this working space, long suction catheters and a variety of instruments to maintain hemostasis should be readily available, including a Harmonic scalpel, bipolar cautery forceps, and clip appliers, ranging in length from 8 to 10 cm to 23 cm.

- The fascia and underlying fibers of the pectoralis major muscle are followed to the clavicle, which is then followed medially. It is important to trace along the course of the clavicle, because this landmark leads the surgeon directly to the medial origin of the sternocleidomastoid muscle.
- Once identified, the fibers of the sternocleidomastoid are outlined superiorly, identifying the division between the medial (sternal; anterior half) and the lateral (clavicular; posterior half) head of the sternocleidomastoid.
- The working space should be created from the clavicular head to just above the omohyoid muscle, which usually correlates with the superior border of the thyroid gland.
- The authors then place the Chung retractor under the sternal head of the sternocleidomastoid and sternohyoid musculature. Once these muscles are elevated,

the surgeon will then find the thyroid lobe, usually covered by the adherent ster-nothyroid muscle.

- As in open surgery, the uppermost fibers of the sternothyroid muscle must also be dissected off the superior pole of the gland.
- Before proceeding to dock the robot, the surgeon should confirm the dimensions of the working space, extending from lateral to medial, from the axilla to across the midline, and from just above the clavicular head to above the omohyoid (Video 1). Without adequate working space, the robotic procedure cannot be effectively or efficiently performed.
- Once the adequacy of the working space is confirmed, the retractor is secured to the table mount, which is placed by the circulating nurse on the contralateral bedpost, at the level of the patient's auricle.

Docking the Robot

Robotic thyroidectomy is an endoscopic neck surgery that provides the surgeon with the ability to dissect the surgical field using time-honored principles of traction and countertraction. This procedure is possible using a binocular stereoendoscope and 3 additional instruments. With these 4 "arms," a surgeon can visualize the surgical anatomy in 3 dimensions, retract, and still use 2 additional instruments for dissection and hemostasis. A binocular camera is placed through the axillary incision with 30° down orientation. Therefore, understanding these relationships is critical to proper docking and setting up of the surgical system to facilitate robotic thyroidectomy. The instruments should enter high so that the surgeon can direct activity without inadvertent trauma to the great vessels, thyroid parenchyma, and nerve. When available, bariatric cannulae can be used for each instrument to allow the robotic arms to be spaced further apart, facilitating a more seamless robotic docking.

Robotic Thyroidectomy

- The authors prefer to start the procedure by first dividing the superior thyroid vascular pedicle.
- Using the 8-mm ProGrasp forceps, the superior thyroid pole is gently retracted caudally but most importantly, out of the tracheoesophageal groove. The gland can then be distinguished from the fibers of the cricothyroid muscle.
- Using the 5-mm Maryland forceps, the pedicle is isolated, then divided with the Harmonic scalpel, close to the gland.
- Along the superior and deep posterolateral aspect of the gland, the parathyroid gland is identified and preserved with its blood supply intact.
- The cervical trachea just below the isthmus should then be identified.

Surgical Note: To facilitate this maneuver, the ProGrasp forceps should be released from above and then placed inferiorly, exerting a cephalad vector of force, opening up this soft tissue plane.

- Thyrothymic and mediastinal veins are divided with the Harmonic scalpel, which allows the surgeon to fully mobilize the inferior aspect of the gland and begin to outline the depth of the tracheoesophageal groove.

Surgical Note: In conventional open thyroid surgery, this determination of "depth" is intuitive. However, in the virtual reconstruction of this surgical anatomy, these relationships may be more difficult to discern even when rendered in high definition. Therefore, as the next step, the robotic surgeon should clearly identify the cervical trachea.

- The middle thyroid vein is ligated with the Harmonic scalpel, followed by the inferior thyroid veins.
- The ProGrasp retractor is then used to retract the thyroid gland out of the tracheoesophageal groove, and the inferior parathyroid gland is identified and preserved.
- Using the fine dissecting Maryland forceps, the recurrent laryngeal nerve is identified and carefully dissected. Branches of the inferior thyroid artery are controlled once the course of the recurrent nerve has been traced.

Surgical Note: Experience with the Harmonic scalpel helps facilitate safe and effective robotic thyroidectomy. The Harmonic scalpel lacks full wristed motion compared with the other robotic instruments, limiting the degrees of freedom with which the surgeon can dissect and possibly creating difficulties during the dissection of the nerve. Furthermore, the robotic surgeon must consider heat generated by the activated blade of the Harmonic scalpel. Therefore, great care should be taken to minimize the risk of thermal injury to the recurrent laryngeal nerve to prevent postoperative neuropraxia.

- After activation, the authors often allow 3 to 5 seconds to pass before coming within 5 to 10 mm of the recurrent laryngeal nerve.
- As the nerve is released from tracheal attachments of the posterior suspensory ligament of Berry, the thyroid gland is removed.
- Telescopic 3-dimensional visualization and precise dissection with the 5-mm Maryland forceps often enable the robotic surgeon to completely remove the thyroid gland.
- The isthmus is then divided using the Harmonic scalpel and the surgery is completed.
- The authors prefer to use a closed suction drain, either through one end of the axillary incision or through a well-camouflaged location within a naturally occurring skin crease.

POSTOPERATIVE MANAGEMENT

Patients generally stay overnight and are discharged from the hospital the morning after the surgery. The drain is often removed on postoperative day 1. However, because of a larger working space compared with open surgery, the risk of postoperative airway compression from hematoma is likely lower than with conventional open surgery. Therefore, discharging patients on the same day of surgery may also be reasonable.

SUPPLEMENTARY DATA

Supplementary data related to this article can be found online at http://dx.doi.org/10.1016/j.otc.2014.03.001.

SUGGESTED READINGS

Holsinger FC, Terris DJ, Kuppersmith RB. Robotic thyroidectomy: operative technique using a transaxillary endoscopic approach without CO2 insufflation. Otolaryngol Clin North Am 2010;43:381–8.

Ikeda Y, Takami H, Sasaki Y, et al. Comparative study of thyroidectomies. Endoscopic surgery versus conventional open surgery. Surg Endosc 2002;19:1741–5.

Kang SW, Jeong JJ, Nam KH, et al. Robot-assisted endoscopic thyroidectomy for thyroid malignancies using a gasless transaxillary approach. J Am Coll Surg 2009; 2009:e1–7.

Kang SW, Jeong JJ, Yun JS, et al. Gasless endoscopic thyroidectomy using transaxillary approach; surgical outcome of 581 patients. Endocr J 2009;56:361–9.

Kang SW, Jeong JJ, Yun JS, et al. Robot-assisted endoscopic surgery for thyroid cancer: experience with the first 100 patients. Surg Endosc 2009;23:2399–406.

Kuppersmith RB, Holsinger FC. Robotic thyroid surgery: an initial experience with North American Patients. Laryngoscope 2010;121(3):521–6.

Lewis CM, Chung WY, Holsinger FC. Feasibility and surgical approach of robotic thyroidectomy without CO2 insufflation. Head Neck 2010;32:121–6.

Yoon JH, Park CH, Chung WY. Gasless endoscopic thyroidectomy via an axillary approach: experience of 30 cases. Surg Laparosc Endosc Percutan Tech 2006;16:226–31.

Transoral Robotic Surgery for Larynx Cancer

Richard V. Smith, MD

KEYWORDS

• Transoral • Robot • Surgery • Larynx • Laryngectomy • Cancer • Cordectomy

KEY POINTS

- Appropriate patient selection, from both a tumor and anatomic standpoint, is the most important consideration in transoral robotic laryngeal surgery.
- The patient must understand the possible complications and limitations of the surgery, and the surgery must be part of a comprehensive plan to manage the cancer.
- The goal should be negative margin surgery and treatment consolidation, attempting unimodal therapy whenever possible.
- En bloc resection, when appropriate, is often possible with this technique.
- It is clearly preferable to perform this surgery before radiation therapy, as radiation complicates the healing and functional outcomes.

Videos of a TORS supraglottic laryngectomy for a T2N0M0 squamous cell carcinoma using the Omniguide CO_2 laser and a TORS total laryngectomy accompany this article at http://www.oto.theclinics.com/

INTRODUCTION

The current techniques of transoral robotic partial and total laryngectomy represent waypoints along a continuum in the development of minimally invasive surgery for laryngeal cancer. The acceptance of transoral robotic surgery (TORS) as a whole, and for the larynx in particular, has been rapid and is based on few clinical data.[1–3] The oncologic basis of this approach comes from the results of transoral laser microsurgical (TLM) resection of larynx cancer, which has an established record of success.[4–8] TORS is a natural extension of the TLM technique. Some argue that TLM is superior, as there are a wider variety of endoscopes and instruments used during the resection, whereas others believe the 3-dimensional high-definition visualization provided by the surgical robot, among other factors, makes TORS a more preferable modality. Increasing experience with TORS techniques have led to decreased

Disclosures: There is nothing to disclose and there are no actual or potential conflicts of interest.
Department of Otorhinolaryngology - Head and Neck Surgery, Albert Einstein College of Medicine, Montefiore Medical Center, 3400 Bainbridge Avenue, Bronx, NY 10467, USA
E-mail address: rsmith@montefiore.org

Otolaryngol Clin N Am 47 (2014) 379–395
http://dx.doi.org/10.1016/j.otc.2014.03.003

complication rates and decreased hospitalization.[9] In addition, TORS management of oropharynx and supraglottic cancers has been shown to result in better short-term and long-term swallowing function in comparison with chemoradiotherapy.[10] This article focuses primarily on TORS supraglottic partial laryngectomy, with some discussion of TORS total laryngectomy and cordectomy. Other laryngeal TORS techniques have been reported, including benign lesion excision and supracricoid partial laryngectomy,[11] but are not discussed here.

TREATMENT GOALS

As with any oncologic surgery, the main goal of treatment is to cure the patient of cancer. A secondary, although equally important, goal in patients with larynx cancer is maximization of their function and quality of life. Successful achievement of cure and preservation of function is aided by TORS partial laryngectomy. Negative margin transoral supraglottic laryngectomy, with selective neck dissection, provides cure rates equivalent to those of chemoradiotherapy, and has the potential to avoid the use of adjuvant radiation, which can result in superior swallowing and speech function while maintaining excellent cure rates.

The overall goals remain the same for primary TORS laryngeal surgery or salvage surgery: tumor eradication with maintenance of the laryngeal functions of speech, swallowing, and breathing. The outcomes and complications are different in the 2 scenarios, with poor wound healing and loss of function being more significant in the salvage setting. Significant dysphagia is more common in the salvage group because of delayed healing and, although rarely required in a primary setting, tracheotomy may be required during the perioperative and healing phase in salvage surgery. Previously irradiated laryngeal tissues have a higher propensity for edema of the residual tissue, which will nearly always resolve over time. In either primary or salvage TORS for laryngeal cancer, swallowing and airway function are excellent in most patients.

PREOPERATIVE PLANNING AND SPECIAL EQUIPMENT

Preoperative planning for any tumor resection is critical. For partial, or total, laryngectomy anatomic imaging is required, with the exception of superficial T1 and select T2 glottic tumors. Standard imaging would include a contrast computed tomography (CT) scan to evaluate the thyroid and cricoid cartilages, the pre-epiglottic and paraglottic spaces, and the cervical lymph nodes. Positron emission tomography in combination with CT is increasingly used, and can help identify disease laterally in the neck in the absence of radiographically positive adenopathy on anatomic imaging. As with all patients with head and neck cancer, a frank discussion with the patient and his or her family of all available treatment modalities is crucial. Evaluation by the appropriate nonsurgical specialists with prospective presentation at a Multidisciplinary Tumor Board is also an important part of the treatment plan.

Special equipment is required for this type of surgery. In addition to the da Vinci Surgical Robot (Intuitive Surgical Systems, Sunnyvale, CA), multiple robotic instruments are important in maximizing operative success. The surgical arms should include a Maryland forceps, Schertel forceps, and Teflon-coated blade-tip electrocautery. A CO_2 fiber laser (or another type of fiber laser) is advantageous when performing TORS on the larynx. The surgical arms should be 5-mm instruments and the endoscope 12 mm if possible. If transoral suturing is planned, 8-mm needle drivers should be used in both arms, as the distal tip of the 8-mm robotic arm articulates in a much shorter radius, facilitating suturing in a confined space. The bedside assistant is responsible for the management of significant hemorrhage from vessels such as the superior laryngeal artery. A laparoscopic articulating clip applier is used for significant vessels, while the robotic cautery or a suction cautery will control the greater part of any intraoperative bleeding. The small or medium clip applier may be used, at the discretion of the surgeon. Laparoscopic peanuts and the Hurd retractor are also useful adjuvants for tissue retraction. Finally, the Feyh-Kastenbauer (FK) retractor system (Gyrus Medical Inc, Maple Grove, MN) is required to maximize exposure options during the surgery. Crowe-Davis and Dingman mouth gags may also be useful.

SPECIAL FEATURES
Patient Selection

Appropriate patient selection is critical for TORS of the larynx, accounting for features of both tumor and patient. As is the case with TLM, establishing appropriate patient expectations are paramount, as there will always be a temporary compromise of swallowing following supraglottic partial laryngectomy. Adequate pulmonary reserve is required to tolerate small amounts of temporary aspiration. In addition, poorly controlled diabetes can impair wound healing after partial laryngectomy.[12] When TORS is used for salvage surgery, one can expect delayed healing and potentially worse functional outcomes.

Tumor stage and extent is an important consideration. Supraglottic tumors, T1 to T4a, may be considered for transoral resection. Supraglottic laryngectomy can be a technically demanding procedure, so those new to the technique should confine themselves to T1 or T2 tumors. Once a surgeon is more experienced, larger tumors can be considered. Neither pre-epiglottic space involvement nor tongue-base involvement are contraindications to TORS resection, provided the exposure is adequate. However, extension into the paraglottic area with vocal-fold immobility (**Fig. 1**) is a contraindication to a TORS supraglottic laryngectomy if electrocautery is used for the dissection, because thermal injury near the glottis area may result in bilateral vocal-fold immobility and the need for a permanent tracheotomy. For this reason, in the author's opinion any TORS glottic surgery should be avoided if electrocautery is used. The development of laser-carrying fibers and manipulators for the robotic arms will facilitate the development and expansion of glottic surgery with TORS. Special consideration should also be undertaken in cases of salvage partial laryngectomy. In addition to poor healing, the tissue planes relied on for margin assessment are much

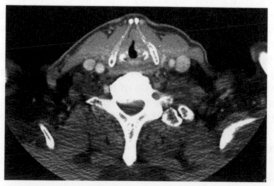

Fig. 1. Axial contrast-enhanced computed tomography of the larynx showing left paraglottic space involvement with tumor. Note absence of fat on the left, with enhancing nodule extending anteriorly on the left.

less obvious, and soft-tissue edema can affect the interaction of the cautery and the tissue, complicating the procedure and the outcomes.

Equipment and anatomic factors are equally important for TORS of the larynx. Current retractor systems have been, for the most part, developed for TLM and not for TORS. The instrumentation required, two 5-mm instruments and a 12-mm telescope, are much more bulky than the TLM instruments. Consequently, instrument conflicts become more significant as one proceeds into the distal pharynx or larynx, as the space becomes more constrained and the instruments begin to cone down. Therefore, maximal mouth opening is essential, precluding the surgery in cases of trismus. In addition, full dentition, particularly the presence of central incisors, can significantly impede exposure. Anterior laryngeal positioning also provides a challenge to adequate exposure, although TORS is less limited in this regard than TLM. A narrow posterior mandibular arch also negatively affects the ability to adequately expose the larynx. Adequate exposure is the most important technical feature, and a variety of retractors should be available for every case to maximize exposure. The minimum retractor complement should include a Crowe-Davis and FK retractor system. Multiple blades may be required for any given procedure, and several may need to be assessed before the optimal exposure is obtained. Exposure should be assessed carefully at the staging endoscopy. Staging endoscopy is advised for all patients with laryngeal cancer considering TORS, as a careful endoscopic evaluation of the tumor is required to determine resectability and accessibility.

Patient and Robot Positioning

As with any surgical procedure, proper positioning of patient and equipment is important.

- For TORS in general, the patient should be supine on the operating table with the head positioned 180° from anesthesia, at the foot of the bed.
- The head of the patient should be positioned as far from the base of the bed as possible, either by turning the bed so the head of the patient is at the foot of the bed or sliding the bed away from the foot support to maximize the distance between the head of the patient and the closest part of the operating room table pedestal. This location gives the maximum amount of flexibility for positioning of the robot.
- A shoulder roll is generally not necessary, as it will frequently compromise the anterior/posterior exposure.
- A suture is placed transversely through the anterior midline tongue, perpendicular to the direction of the muscle fibers, to facilitate exposure by tongue traction. Care must be taken to avoid compression of the tongue between the teeth and the retractor blade during the surgery.
- Once the retractor has been positioned and held in place with a self-retaining arm, the lips are coated with Lacrilube to minimize trauma and desiccation.
- The robot is brought in from the side of the bed, the right side at the author's institution, at a 30° angle from the long axis of the bed.
- In general, 2 robotic arms are used and brought in from the lateral aspects of the mouth, with the camera placed centrally.
- The arms are carefully positioned to avoid conflict between each other and the cannulas guiding the arms are placed in the mouth at the fulcrum point of the arm, designated by the wide dark stripe on the cannula (**Fig. 2**).
- The instruments are advanced into the robotic arms under visualization, and the resection begins.
- For most laryngeal TORS procedure, the 30° endoscope is used facing up.

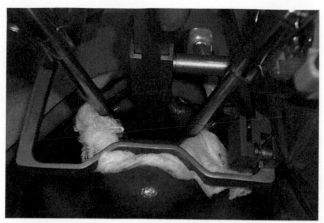

Fig. 2. Intraoral relationship of the FK retractor and the robotic arms. Note the wide black bands at the oral commissure denoting the rotational axis of the instrument. The endoscope is not inserted in this photo.

PROCEDURE
Supraglottic Laryngectomy

The dissection for a supraglottic laryngectomy begins superiorly, in all cases, after adequate exposure and visualization has been confirmed.

Surgical Note: *The main limitations are usually in the anterior/posterior exposure of the larynx, owing to either radiation changes or anatomic features of the patient.*

The following technical description is that of a complete supraglottic laryngectomy. The extent of the dissection will depend on the extent and location of the tumor. An example is presented in the accompanying video (Video 1), in which a complete TORS supraglottic laryngectomy is performed with the CO_2 laser.

- The dissection is initiated either at the anterior aspect of the vallecula or the lateral aspect of the pharyngoepiglottic fold (**Fig. 3**).
- This dissection should be carried to the inner surface of the hyoid to facilitate complete removal of the pre-epiglottic space.
- The superior laryngeal vascular bundle is predictably encountered fairly early in the dissection of the lateral pharyngoepiglottic fold. These vessels should be taken prospectively and controlled with 5-mm vascular clips using a laparoscopic clip applier.
- If the vessel is transected before it is clipped, it should be stabilized with the robotic forceps and subsequently clipped. It should not be managed with cautery.
- The dissection proceeds anteriorly and laterally to resect the pre-epiglottic space in continuity with the tumor (**Fig. 4**).
- The aryepiglottic folds are then transected superior and lateral to the arytenoid, incising obliquely to transect the posterior vestibular fold and enter the ventricle (**Fig. 5**).
- The transection continues anteriorly at the ventricular apex until the petiole and anterior commissure are encountered (**Fig. 6**).
- The pre-epiglottic dissection is connected to the transection inferior to the epiglottic petiole to allow removal of the specimen. If necessary, division of the specimen into quadrants is performed to improve exposure and visualization of the dissection planes.

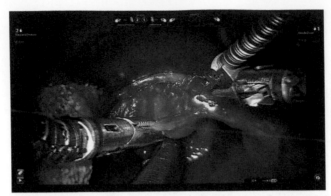

Fig. 3. Lateral pharyngoepiglottic fold cut to begin a TORS supraglottic laryngectomy. The left instrument, Schertel forceps, is grasping and retracting the epiglottis while the right directs the laser.

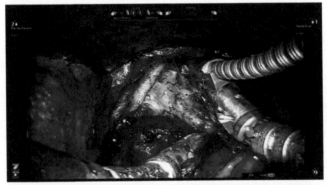

Fig. 4. Anterior dissection of the pre-epiglottic fat at the thyroid ala. The left thyroid ala is visible and the left robotic arm is grasping and retracting the pre-epiglottic fat.

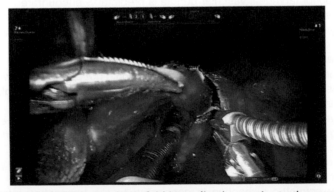

Fig. 5. Incision of the right aryepiglottic fold immediately superior to the corniculate cartilage. This incision will be taken anterior and inferior to enter the right ventricle. The left robotic arm is grasping the epiglottis and retracting it anterolaterally. The armored endotracheal tube is visualized entering the larynx.

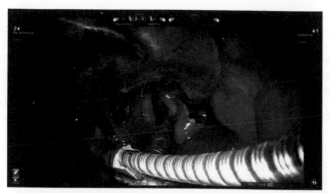

Fig. 6. The anterior cuts, at the level of the false vocal fold bilaterally, are shown immediately before connecting them at the petiole with the anterior pre-epiglottic dissection.

- Hemostasis is obtained and the area irrigated.
- Margins can be taken as necessary to assess the adequacy of resection.

Surgical Note: Dissection into the inferior paraglottic space may result in immobility of the ipsilateral vocal fold, owing to scar fixation; this should not be undertaken with electrocautery.

- Use of a laser fiber may allow a limited paraglottic resection as required, but should be avoided bilaterally.
- An arytenoid may be resected if necessary oncologically, but should be avoided if possible, as postoperative swallowing function will be compromised. Local flap reconstruction should be considered in such cases. This technique is well described by Dziegielewski and Ozer.[13]

Total Laryngectomy

TORS total laryngectomy is a procedure in evolution, and limited case series have been published. To date, this procedure has been primarily in cases of salvage laryngectomy not requiring concurrent neck dissection. Careful patient selection is required, as the exposure considerations are more pertinent to this procedure given the dissection deeper within the pharynx. This procedure is technically demanding, and should not be considered if the surgeon is not experienced in transoral tumor surgery.

The accompanying video demonstrates the technique (Video 2).

- The procedure begins with a transcutaneous approach to the trachea to secure the airway under local anesthesia.
- The stomal incision is outlined between the cricoid cartilage and suprasternal notch, the skin of the stomal site is excised, and dissection of the pretracheal tissue is completed with division of the thyroid isthmus.
- The anterior trachea is exposed from the cricoid to the fourth tracheal ring, and the trachea is entered between the second and third rings.
- An anode endotracheal tube is placed and general endotracheal anesthesia initiated, after which paratracheal dissection, either unilateral or bilateral, is completed through the stomal opening.
- The posterior wall of the trachea is then incised and the posterior tissues are mobilized superiorly, separating the remaining superior trachea from the esophagus.

- The anterior half of the trachea is then matured to the inferior stomal incision, and the remainder of the procedure, with the exception of closing the superior half of the stoma and insertion of a closed suction drain, is completed transorally.
- The resection begins by incising the lateral pharyngoepiglottic fold and anterior vallecula in the standard fashion used for endoscopic supraglottic laryngectomy.
- The hyoid bone is dissected free from the pre-epiglottic tissues, maintaining the integrity of the fascial compartment containing the pre-epiglottic fat, and this plane of dissection is continued inferiorly to expose the superior border of the thyroid cartilage (**Fig. 7**).
- Once identified, the thyroid ala is mobilized posteriorly, leaving the outer thyroid perichondrium intact.
- The anterior pyriform sinus mucosa is incised and the lateral pyriform mucosa is mobilized (**Fig. 8**).

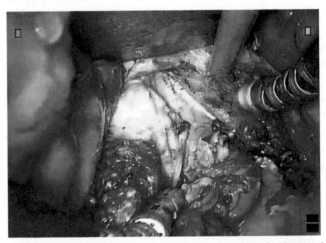

Fig. 7. The superior aspect of the right thyroid ala is visualized. The suction cautery is retracting the hyoid bone anteriorly and the pre-epiglottic tissue is intact medially.

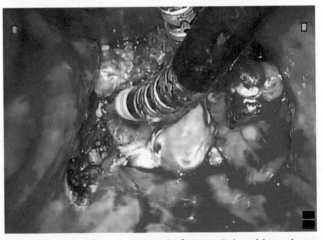

Fig. 8. The left deep pyriform sinus is exposed after medial and lateral mucosal cuts. The electrocautery tip is exposing the pyriform, and the left arytenoid is visualized medially and posteriorly.

- Transection of the superior laryngeal suspensory ligament facilitates access to the constrictor muscles, which are then dissected (**Fig. 9**).
- The muscles are then sharply divided, along with the remaining fascia separating the intraoral dissection from the stomal dissection. At this point the only area preventing removal of the larynx is the postcricoid area.
- The postcricoid mucosal cut is made under direct transoral visualization, providing appropriate margins for the tumor, and the remainder of the specimen is dissected.
- The larynx is then fully mobilized and removed transorally (**Fig. 10**).
- Closure of the wound is then performed.
- All surfaces are irrigated and hemostasis is assured, after which the mucosal incision is closed with several running 3-0 Vicryl sutures.
- The pharynx is closed primarily with a single horizontal suture line (**Fig. 11**).

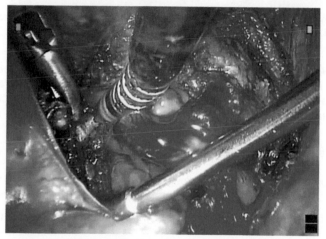

Fig. 9. The constrictor muscles are incised at their attachment to the left posterior thyroid ala. The left arm of the robot is lateralizing the upper left thyroid ala for better exposure.

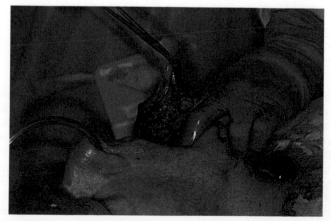

Fig. 10. The larynx is removed transorally.

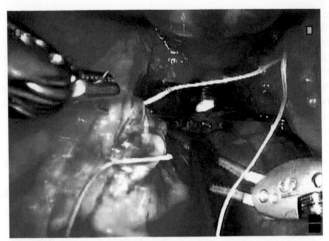

Fig. 11. The mucosal incisions are sutured under direct visualization. The lateral left aspect of the wound being closed after removal of the larynx.

Surgical Note: As the integrity of the strap muscles is maintained, if the mucosa is not sufficient to close to itself primarily, the inferior and lateral mucosal surfaces may be closed to the strap muscles in a U-shaped configuration, allowing the central component to heal by secondary intention, as is currently the standard for endoscopic resections.

- The area is again irrigated and inspected from the stoma to confirm a watertight closure.
- A suction drain is then placed through a separate stab incision into the external compartment, and the stomal suturing is completed to finish the procedure.

The technique of robotic total laryngectomy is well illustrated by Smith.[14]

POTENTIAL COMPLICATIONS AND MANAGEMENT

The potential complications of this surgery can be broken down into those related to the robot and those related to the tumor removal.

Standard complications apply to the tumor removal and include:

- Bleeding
- Airway compromise
- Swallowing dysfunction
- Fistula

Hemorrhage is the most feared of the complications, because these patients usually do not have a tracheotomy in place and a significant, acute bleeding episode could obstruct the airway in addition to hemodynamic changes. The most effective management of a postoperative hemorrhage is prevention and avoidance of perioperative antithrombotic medications.[15] A detailed understanding of the vascular anatomy, from inside to out, is critical for successful transoral laryngeal supraglottic or total laryngectomy. The large vessels should be prospectively identified and must be clipped, not cauterized, to minimize the risk of a significant postoperative hemorrhage.

Airway compromise is rarely an issue after the tumor has been removed, unless there is a significant amount of redundant and edematous tissue left in place following the resection. This residue should be managed at the time of the resection, and more likely is present in a previously irradiated patient.

Aspiration and swallowing abnormalities are the norm following supraglottic laryngectomy; all patients should have a formal swallowing evaluation, with maneuvers, before initiating oral feeding.

Fistula is uncommon and most likely if concurrent extensive neck dissection is performed; if noted intraoperatively, a fistula should be managed with local tissue coverage.

Other unusual complications, such as skin necrosis from transoral dissection of the subcutaneous tissues,[16] have been reported.

Complications related to the robot are uncommon and include:

- Dental injury
- Mucosal laceration
- Device malfunction

These problems can be avoided by careful placement of the robotic arms and focused attention of the bedside assistant. Device malfunction is very unlikely, but backup robotic arms should be available.

POSTPROCEDURAL CARE AND RECOVERY

The same postoperative care used for open or TLM procedures is used for TORS supraglottic or total laryngectomy. For supraglottic laryngectomy, postoperative humidification, proton-pump inhibitors, antibiotics, and cervical wound care is routine. As noted earlier, initially nasogastric feeding is used, followed by a careful assessment of swallowing by a speech/swallow therapist. The initiation of oral intake should be supervised and use whichever swallowing maneuvers are effective. Early postoperative resumption of oral intake is expected in most of these patients. Care for the total laryngectomy patient is not different to that for an open total laryngectomy, consisting of nasogastric feeding, stomal care, humidification, antibiotics, and cervical wound care.

OUTCOMES AND CLINICAL RESULTS IN THE LITERATURE

There are limited long-term data on the oncologic results of TORS in general, and particularly TORS of the larynx. Most studies have presented varied primary sites, predominantly oropharynx, and have discussed complication and safety issues, short-term quality of life, and short-term oncologic results. Functional results have focused on swallowing function and tracheotomy rates. In a study for the University of Alabama involving 29 of 36 patients undergoing successful TORS for head and neck cancer, 10 patients had laryngeal cancer.[17] Seven of the 10 had a successful resection, and 4 of these 7 were extubated at the completion of the procedure. The remainder had planned intubation (2) or emergent reintubation (1), and all were subsequently successfully extubated. However, 6 of the 7 required prolonged tube feeding. Park and colleagues[18] recently reviewed their experience with 141 patients managed with TORS and included 36 patients with laryngeal cancer. Unlike other series, most of their laryngeal patients (26) had glottic cancers. All patients who had cancer underwent tracheotomy, regardless of tumor site. Specific results on decannulation and swallowing function were not presented. The 2-year disease-free survival for the entire cohort was 91%, with that of the patients with laryngeal cancer not reported independently. An earlier analysis by the same group looking specifically at laryngeal and hypopharyngeal cancers noted all 5 laryngeal patients to be decannulated by postoperative day 8 and to resume oral feeding by postoperative day 7.[19]

TORS of the larynx has been limited by several factors. The current retractor systems more easily expose the oropharynx, instrument conflicts increase the further the lesion is from the oral opening, and the limited instrumentation further complicates the procedure. Glottic surgery was first described in a canine model,[20] and has subsequently been reported in humans.[18,21] Most surgeons have been hesitant to perform glottic surgery in the absence of an integrated robotic laser instrument, fearing the potential collateral damage from monopolar electrocautery. Kayhan and colleagues[21] first reported a series of 10 patients undergoing TORS cordectomy with electrocautery. All were stage T1 and achieved negative margins, and 9 were extubated immediately postoperatively and began oral alimentation on the day of surgery. One required a temporary tracheotomy and nasogastric tube. The 26 patients with glottic cancer reported by Park and colleagues[18] also all underwent cordectomy with monopolar electrocautery. Voice results and larynx function have not been reported in either series, so comparison with TLM approaches and radiation-therapy voice results cannot be performed. One must remain concerned about vocal function in the absence of a laser, although this may soon change as laser couplers have been developed by several companies, including Lumenis and Omniguide.[22,23]

There are still serious technical limitations to TORS of the larynx. De Virgilio and colleagues[24] have described their techniques to optimize laryngeal and hypopharyngeal exposure during TORS. This approach was based on TORS for 22 hypopharyngeal cancers, 19 glottic cancers, and 7 supraglottic cancers. These investigators recommend the following: (1) trial the FK retractor system and 30° telescope for exposure during the initial diagnostic laryngoscopy; (2) use intraoperative muscle relaxants; (3) routinely perform tracheotomy before the TORS; (4) use the 30° robotic endoscope positioned as far from the operative site as feasible; (5) position the 30° scope at the posterior pharyngeal wall at an acute angle; (6) retract the tongue anteriorly; (7) perform an ipsilateral epiglottectomy for pyriform sinus lesions. Their exposure outcomes were mixed, with 4 laryngeal patients deemed "good" exposure, 21 "fair," and 1 "poor." Those with hypopharyngeal cancers more frequently had poor or fair exposure. Unlike open cases, the current instrumentation for TORS laryngeal surgery continues to affect procedures.

Most reports of TORS for laryngeal resection have concerned supraglottic tumors, the functional and oncologic results of which are presented in **Table 1**. Initial descriptions were published by Solares and Strome,[25] who performed TORS supraglottic laryngectomy in 3 patients, while Weinstein and colleagues[26] reported their series of 3 successful TORS supraglottic laryngectomies. TORS supraglottic laryngectomy came about at a time when TLM supraglottic partial laryngectomy had gained oncologic acceptance among many head and neck surgeons. Therefore several centers began using this technique, believing that the 3-dimensional visualization, angled view and working space, and relative ease of surgical technique make this a desirable alternative to TLM supraglottic laryngectomy. The feasibility of TORS supraglottic laryngectomy was assessed by Alon and colleagues,[16] who used this technique in 7 patients with T1 to T3 lesions using the FK retractor with the laryngeal blade. Four of their patients received tracheotomy, which remained in place for a range of 4 days to permanent, and 5 patients had prolonged tube feedings. Two had gastrostomies (time not reported) and 3 had prolonged nasogastric tube placements (38–56 days). Two of their patients with N2 neck disease, both of whom had gastrostomy tubes and one of whom had a permanent tracheotomy tube, underwent adjuvant radiotherapy. The follow-up was too brief to evaluate survival.

Table 1
Results of transoral robotic resection for supraglottic cancer

Authors,[Ref.] Year	No. of Patients	Initial T1/T2 (%)	Positive Margins (%)	Perioperative Tracheotomy (%)	Gastrostomy (%)	Complications	Adjuvant Therapy (%)	2-Year DSS (%)
Weinstein et al,[26] 2007	3	67 (2/3)	0	NA	0[a]	None	33 (1/3)	NA
Ozer et al,[27] 2013	13	85 (11/13)	0	0	8 (1/13)	None	15 (2/13)	NA
Olsen et al,[28] 2012	9	78 (7/9)	0	78 (7/9)	44 (4/9)	1 supraglottic stenosis	67 (6/9)	88
Park et al,[29] 2013	16	75 (12/16)	12 (2/16)	100[b]	0	None	50 (8/16)	91
Mendelsohn et al,[30] 2013	18	72 (13/16)	0	0	0	5, not specified	50 (9/18)	100

This table represents current publications describing supraglottic TORS. Several publications were omitted owing to either low numbers of successful surgeries or patients being included in the series reported here.

Abbreviations: DSS, disease-specific survival; NA, not available.
[a] Routine use of prolonged nasogastric tubes.
[b] Routine use of perioperative tracheotomy, all patients decannulated.

Subsequent studies have presented larger, but still small, patient series, and have shown good results. However, interestingly there is a significant institutional bias to the use of tracheotomy and/or gastrostomy tubes. The Korean group remains the only published group to routinely perform tracheotomy[29] and, in general, most surgeons see these techniques as a way to avoid routine tracheotomy and feeding-tube placement, both of which have a negative impact on quality of life. Functional recovery is excellent, with some investigators instituting oral feeding on postoperative day 1.[27] Tumor stage has been predominantly early-stage disease (T1 or T2), but T3 lesions, based on pre-epiglottic extension, are also amenable to this technique. Mendelsohn has found tumor stage to be an important predictor of functional recovery, with early T stage (pT1/pT2) having a statistically significant earlier return to swallowing, both liquids and solids, than late T stage (pT3/T4).[30] This finding is intuitive given that larger surgical defects result in greater sacrifice of compensatory structures. Female gender, simultaneous neck dissection, and vocal-fold hypomobility were also found to have significance.

Survival data have been limited for TORS of the larynx. The mean follow-up for all series has been less than 3 years, significantly limiting the generalizability of the oncologic results. Mendelsohn and colleagues[30] have reported 2-year outcomes in their 18 patients with a mean follow-up of 28 months. Their locoregional control, disease-specific survival, and overall survival was 83%, 100%, and 89%, respectively. Three patients had recurrence in the neck, 1 of whom only had a sentinel node biopsy, and there were 4 distant failures. Half of their patients received adjuvant chemotherapy and radiation therapy for advanced neck disease. Park and colleagues[29] have reported 16 patients with a mean follow-up of 20 months and report a 2-year disease-free survival rate of 91%, although only 2 patients enrolled had a follow-up of more than 20 months. Half of their patients underwent adjuvant therapy as well, 19% with radiation only (for pT3 disease) and 31% with chemotherapy and radiation (2 for positive margins and 3 for extracapsular nodal spread). These investigators also compared their TORS supraglottic laryngectomy patients with a matched cohort of open supraglottic laryngectomy patients and found earlier decannulation, earlier oral feeding, and shorter hospitalization in the TORS group.

There has been a wide variability in the application of adjuvant therapy. Most often the adjuvant therapy is used for advanced nodal disease rather than positive margins. The poor prognosis associated with extracapsular spread in the human papillomavirus–negative patient or 3 or more positive nodes can justify this approach. In the author's center, the central structures are shielded from full-dose radiotherapy to maximize pharyngeal and laryngeal function. The use of adjuvant therapy, however, is not without consequence, as long-term functional complications following TORS, either prolonged tracheotomy or gastrostomy, are often present only in this treatment group.[28] The goal of surgical therapy in these patients should be avoidance of adjuvant therapy if at all possible, using the TORS and neck dissection as unimodal therapy. If adjuvant therapy is known to be necessary at the onset, one must carefully assess the benefits and risks of adding surgery to the treatment plan.

TORS total laryngectomy is a new extension of this operative modality. Although only 2 series of patients have been reported thus far, the results are promising.[31,32] Salvage surgery is the main indication for this procedure at present, and access remains the limiting factor. The pliability of laryngeal and pharyngeal structures is often decreased following chemotherapy and radiation, and the pharyngeal operative field is often reduced from local tissue contracture, fibrosis, and stenosis. Of particular concern for this procedure is the placement of a tracheotomy before the procedure. Low tracheotomy has a detrimental effect on TORS total laryngectomy, and should be carefully assessed preoperatively.[31] Dowthwaite and colleagues[32] recommend exposure with the FK retractor at the time of tumor endoscopy to maximize the opportunity for successful TORS laryngectomy. The challenging exposure is often inferiorly in the pyriform sinus and postcricoid region. This situation can be managed with a slight extension of the stomal incision, in conjunction with the transoral robotic incisions, to complete a more difficult total laryngectomy with a hybrid approach, still using minimally invasive techniques. Although it is a technically challenging procedure, TORS total laryngectomy holds the advantage of limited tissue manipulation during a narrow-field laryngectomy in the recurrence setting. This approach may reduce fistula rates and minimize stricture, given maintenance of the surrounding structures. Its success is also predicated on the ability to limit lateral neck dissection in these patients, addressing level VI during the TORS laryngectomy and leaving levels II to IV undissected.[33,34] At present, the indications for TORS laryngectomy remain undefined.

SUMMARY

TORS of the larynx is an effective and safe method to manage laryngeal cancer in the primary and salvage setting. The challenges are related to equipment and patient-specific anatomic access. If a TLM approach is appropriate for a given supraglottic tumor, most likely a TORS approach will also be appropriate. The magnified angled view, facile instrument motion, and ability to suture deep within the pharynx are benefits of this approach, whereas instrumentation and access are limitations. Instrumentation and access can be expected to improve with the development of new robots and retractors designed for TORS. As more surgeons gain experience with this technique, some of these limitations may be eliminated. The concept of transoral partial laryngectomy has been well validated through the use of TLM techniques, and there is no reason to assume that the results will be any different for TORS, provided the surgeon adheres to the standard principles of transoral resection (TORS or TLM).

SUPPLEMENTARY DATA

Supplementary data related to this article can be found online at http://dx.doi.org/10.1016/j.otc.2014.03.003.

REFERENCES

1. Ceruse P, Lallemant B, Moriniere S, et al. Transoral minimally invasive robotic surgery for carcinoma of the pharynx and the larynx: a new approach. Anticancer Drugs 2011;22:591–5.
2. Genden EM, O'Malley BW, Weinstein GS, et al. Transoral robotic surgery: role in management of upper aerodigestive tract tumors. Head Neck 2010;34:886–93.
3. Hans S, Badoual C, Gorphe P, et al. Transoral robotic surgery for head and neck carcinomas. Eur Arch Otorhinolaryngol 2012;269:1979–84.
4. Motta G, Esposito E, Motta S, et al. CO_2 laser surgery in the treatment of glottis cancer. Head Neck 2005;27:566–74.
5. Peretti G, Piazza C, Cocco D, et al. Transoral CO_2 laser treatment for Tis-T3 glottic cancer: the University of Brescia experience on 595 patients. Head Neck 2010; 32:977–83.
6. Iro H, Waldfahrer F, Altendorf-Hofmann A, et al. Transoral laser surgery of supraglottic cancer: follow-up of 141 patients. Arch Otolaryngol Head Neck Surg 1998; 124:1245–50.

7. Motta G, Esposito E, Testa D, et al. CO_2 laser treatment of supraglottic cancer. Head Neck 2004;26:442–6.
8. Bussu F, Almadori G, De Corso E, et al. Endoscopic horizontal partial laryngectomy by CO_2 laser in the management of supraglottic squamous cell carcinoma. Head Neck 2009;31:1196–206.
9. White HN, Frederick J, Zimmerman T, et al. Learning curve for transoral robotic surgery: a 4 year analysis. JAMA Otolaryngol Head Neck Surg 2013;139:564–7.
10. More YI, Tsue TT, Girod DA, et al. Functional swallowing outcomes following transoral robotic surgery vs primary chemoradiotherapy in patients with advanced-stage oropharynx and supraglottis cancers. JAMA Otolaryngol Head Neck Surg 2013;139:43–8.
11. Vural E, Tulunay-Ugur OE, Suen JY. Transoral robotic supracricoid partial laryngectomy with cartilaginous framework preservation. J Robot Surg 2010;6: 363–6.
12. Vilaseca-Gonzalez I, Bernal-Sprekelsen M, Blanch-Alejandro J-L, et al. Complications in transoral CO_2 laser surgery for carcinoma of the larynx and hypopharynx. Head Neck 2003;25:382–8.
13. Dziegielewski PT, Ozer E. Transoral robotic surgery: supraglottic laryngectomy. Operative Techniques in Otolaryngology 2013;24:86–91.
14. Smith RV. Transoral robotic total laryngectomy. Operative Techniques Otolaryngol 2013;24:92–8.
15. Asher SA, White HN, Kejner AE, et al. Hemorrhage after transoral robotic-assisted surgery. Otolaryngol Head Neck Surg 2013;149:112–7.
16. Alon EE, Kasperbauer JL, Olsen KD, et al. Feasibility of transoral robotic-assisted supraglottic laryngectomy. Head Neck 2012;34:225–9.
17. Boudreaux BA, Rosenthal EL, Magnuson JS, et al. Robot-assisted surgery for upper aerodigestive tract neoplasms. Arch Otolaryngol Head Neck Surg 2009;135: 397–401.
18. Park YM, Kim WS, Byeon HK, et al. Clinical outcomes of transoral robotic surgery for head and neck tumors. Ann Otol Rhinol Laryngol 2013;122:73–84.
19. Park YM, Lee WJ, Lee JG, et al. Transoral robotic surgery (TORS) in laryngeal and hypopharyngeal cancer. J Laparoendosc Adv Surg Tech A 2009;19:361–8.
20. O'Malley BW, Weinstein GS, Hockstein NG. Transoral robotic surgery (TORS): glottic microsurgery in a canine model. J Voice 2006;20:263–8.
21. Kayhan FT, Kaya KH, Sayin I. Transoral robotic cordectomy for early glottic carcinoma. Ann Otol Rhinol Laryngol 2012;121:497–502.
22. Remacle M, Matar N, Lawson G, et al. Combining a new CO_2 laser wave guide with transoral robotic surgery: a feasibility on four patients with malignant tumors. Eur Arch Otorhinolaryngol 2010;269:1833–7.
23. Desai SC, Sung CK, Jang DW, et al. Transoral robotic surgery using a carbon dioxide flexible laser for tumors of the upper aerodigestive tract. Laryngoscope 2008;118:2187–9.
24. De Virgilio A, Park YM, Kim WS, et al. How to optimize laryngeal and hypopharyngeal exposure in transoral robotic surgery. Auris Nasus Larynx 2013;40: 312–9.
25. Solares CA, Strome M. Transoral robot-assisted CO_2 laser supraglottic laryngectomy: experimental and clinical data. Laryngoscope 2007;117:817–20.
26. Weinstein GS, O'Malley BW, Snyder W, et al. Transoral robotic surgery: supraglottic partial laryngectomy. Ann Otol Rhinol Laryngol 2007;116:19–23.
27. Ozer E, Alvarez B, Kakarala K, et al. Clinical outcomes of transoral robotic supraglottic laryngectomy. Head Neck 2013;35:1158–61.

28. Olsen SM, Moore EJ, Koch CA, et al. Transoral robotic surgery for supraglottic squamous cell carcinoma. Am J Otolaryngol 2012;33:379–84.
29. Park YM, Kim WS, Byeon HK, et al. Surgical techniques and treatment outcomes of transoral robotic supraglottic partial laryngectomy. Laryngoscope 2013;123: 670–7.
30. Mendelsohn AH, Remacle M, Van Der Vorst S, et al. Outcomes following transoral robotic surgery: supraglottic laryngectomy. Laryngoscope 2012;123:208–14.
31. Smith RV, Schiff BA, Sarta C, et al. Transoral robotic total laryngectomy. Laryngoscope 2012;123:678–82.
32. Dowthwaite S, Nichols AC, Yoo J, et al. Transoral robotic total laryngectomy: report of 3 cases. Head Neck 2013;35:E338–42.
33. Koss SL, Russell MD, Leem TH, et al. Occult nodal disease in patients with failed laryngeal preservation undergoing surgical salvage. Laryngoscope 2014;124(2): 421–8.
34. Basheeth N, O'Leary G, Sheahan P. Elective neck dissection for N0 neck during salvage total laryngectomy: findings, complications, and oncological outcome. JAMA Otolaryngol Head Neck Surg 2013;139:790–6.

Transoral Robotic Sleep Surgery
The Obstructive Sleep Apnea–Hypopnea Syndrome

Julia A. Crawford, MD[a], Filippo Montevechi, MD[b],
Claudio Vicini, MD[b], J. Scott Magnuson, MD[a],*

KEYWORDS

- TORS • Apnea • Sleep-disordered breathing • Sleep medicine

KEY POINTS

- Obstructive sleep apnea–hypopnea syndrome is a heterogeneous disease.
- Gold-standard therapy is continuous positive airway pressure; however, in patients who cannot tolerate this treatment, surgery may be a feasible alternative.
- Transoral robotic surgery (TORS) offers a minimally invasive, well-visualized approach to the base of the tongue.
- Early data looking at surgical success for TORS base-of-tongue resection is encouraging.

INTRODUCTION

Obstructive sleep apnea–hypopnea syndrome (OSAHS) is a common disorder that affects 2% to 4% of the adult population.[1] It is a serious social health problem with significant implications for a patient's quality of life as well as for his or her long-term health.[2] It has been consistently shown to cause a multitude of neurobehavioral issues as well as to be an independent risk factor for cardiopulmonary derangements that significantly increase the risk of death.[3]

The gold standard for treatment remains continuous positive airway pressure (CPAP). However, there are patients who are not able to tolerate this device and require an alternative treatment. Surgery for OSAHS has been criticized because of lack of evidence supporting its efficacy and the heterogeneous results in the published outcomes. Its effectiveness as a viable treatment option was further questioned by a

Disclosure: Dr Magnuson: Lumenis, Intuitive Surgical and Medrobotics Corporation.
[a] Head and Neck Surgery Center of Florida, Celebration Health, Florida Hospital, Suite 305, 410 Celebration Place, Celebration, FL 34747, USA; [b] Special Surgery Department, Otolaryngology-Head and Neck & Oral Surgery Unit, University of Pavia in Forlì, Morgagni Pierantoni Hospital, Via Carlo Forlanini, 34, FL 47100, Italy
* Corresponding author.
E-mail address: scott.magnuson@flhosp.org

Otolaryngol Clin N Am 47 (2014) 397–406
http://dx.doi.org/10.1016/j.otc.2014.03.004
0030-6665/14/$ – see front matter © 2014 Elsevier Inc. All rights reserved.

oto.theclinics.com

large meta-analysis that showed that uvulopalatopharyngoplasty was effective in less than 50% of cases.[4] However, much of the criticism stems from the significant variation in the surgical options available with a lack of consistency in the reporting of outcomes. Additionally, interpretation of the available literature is problematic because of the different apnea-hypopnea index (AHI) criteria for investigation and different AHI thresholds for defining surgical success or improvement.[1]

Surgical approaches range from procedures that increase or stabilize the airway by removing or repositioning tissue to procedures that completely bypass the site of airway collapse, such as tracheostomy.[2] OSAHS is an incredibly complex heterogeneous disorder that requires a thorough assessment before planning intervention. This ensures that the particular level of collapse is addressed on an individual patient basis.

The concept of transoral robotic surgery (TORS) as a treatment of OSAHS was first introduced in 2009 by Vicini and colleagues[5] in their feasibility report looking at the treatment of hypertrophy of the tongue base. Since then, it has been shown to be an effective treatment option for both solely base-of-tongue procedures and when combined with multi-level surgery.

TORS has the ability to overcome the issues with surgical access that had previously hampered surgical treatment options. It has become increasingly understood that tongue base anatomy may play a more important role than previously thought in the pathophysiology of OSAHS. The robot system allows for high-quality endoscopic optics for improved visualization with three-dimensional (3D) depth perception and robotic instrumentation. These instruments have 6° of freedom and 90° of articulation that allows for superior dexterity and precision.[6]

TREATMENT GOALS

In sleep apnea surgery, the criterion for success is not necessarily polysomnographic cure.[7] Although this seems counterintuitive, curing a patient of sleep apnea is not the goal. The goal is achieving either a reduction in AHI scores and/or an improvement in clinical symptomatology. The argument surrounding surgery for OSAHS should be taken in the context of whether the gold-standard treatment can be applied at all times. That is, if a patient wears CPAP for only 4 hours a night, is this really better than a partial cure that is applied throughout the night?[7]

The increase in mortality from cardiovascular risk factors for sleep apnea is in patients in the moderate to severe range. If surgery reduces a moderate or severe sleep apnea patient to a mild sleep apnea patient, although this is not a polysomnographic cure, it is likely to significantly reduce their neurocognitive and cardiopulmonary risk factors.[8–11] If this is achieved in the context of improving their symptoms of daytime sleepiness and snoring, the patient has benefited from the intervention.

In most of the published series, the treatment goals are broken down into surgical cure and surgical response. A surgical cure is defined as a decrease in preoperative AHI of at least 50% and a postoperative AHI of less than 20 events per hour. A surgical response is defined as a reduction from the preoperative AHI of at least 50%.[12]

In terms of the contribution that TORS makes to the sleep surgeon's armamentarium, TORS allows the surgeon to perform procedures that otherwise are done only through an open approach, which usually results in significant morbidity and decreased quality of life.[13]

Essentially, the treatment goal remains not only a significant reduction in AHI but also an improvement in the quality-of-life scores as documented by their Epworth Sleepiness Scale and Snoring Severity Scale which is, perhaps, of even more worth.

PATIENT SELECTION
Indications

The chief indication for surgery in OSAHS is that the patient has failed a trial of the gold-standard treatment, CPAP, because he or she is noncompliant or cannot tolerate the device. Typically, the patient should have polysomnographic evidence of moderate to severe OSAHS in addition to daytime somnolence as documented through the Epworth Sleepiness Scale.[7] For TORS-specific surgery, there should be significant contribution to obstruction at the base of the tongue. This is determined either by awake nasopharyngoscopy with the appropriate maneuvers or by drug-induced sleep endoscopy.

Contraindications

Contraindications for TORS are classified as patient compliance, patient anatomy, and medical comorbidities. The gold-standard treatment of sleep apnea is CPAP therapy. If the patient is compliant with this therapy, surgical intervention is discouraged.

The anatomy of the patient must also be amendable to access with the robot. A degree of trismus or limited mobility of the neck may make the base of the tongue inaccessible. Significant micrognathia and macroglossia may also limit the exposure for TORS procedures, although they may not necessarily make it impossible.[13] Dynamic compression of the lateral airway from soft tissue is a relative contraindication because TORS essentially addresses anterior-posterior collapse of the airway.

Because surgery for OSAHS is a second-line therapy, careful thought must be directed toward the potential risks the patient may face from an anesthetic. An American Society of Anesthesiologists score greater than 2 with particular reference to significant or unstable cardiovascular disease or the need for anticoagulation must be treated with caution.

PREOPERATIVE PLANNING

The preoperative workup is essential for adequately determining the optimum treatment plan for the patient. In those who have failed treatment with CPAP or other devices, a thorough assessment must be undertaken to ensure that their anatomy is amenable to surgery. This should help to ensure that only patients who have a chance of improvement from surgery are offered treatment and that the correct level of obstruction is targeted.

This workup should begin with a targeted sleep history in which the patient and the patient's significant other are involved. Pertinent points to include in this assessment are a snoring history, rhinologic or allergy history, and any history of single-vehicle accidents because patients with OSAHS may have twofold to threefold increased rate of traffic accidents.[9,14,15]

Specific to the OSAHS examination, the body mass index and neck circumference should be noted. Retrognathia or mandibular hypoplasia resulting in malocclusion or a high-arched palate should be noted. The oral tongue size, assessed with a modified Mallampati score, should be noted in addition to the length of the uvula and soft palate. The size of the tonsils, based on a Friedman grading system should also be recorded.

Nasopharyngoscopy identifies septal deviation, enlarged turbinates, inflamed nasal mucosa, and/or adenoid hypertrophy. Additionally, inspection of the hypopharynx allows for characterization of the epiglottis and the volume of hypertrophy of the base of the tongue. Müller and Woodson hypotonic maneuvers are performed in erect and supine positions to ascertain the level of collapse and help determine a targeted approach for treatment.

The preoperative assessment should also include general medical health with particular focus on the relevant comorbidities, including cardiac issues.

RELEVANT ANATOMY

The base of the tongue has a rich vascular supply from the lingual artery. Significant vessels are located laterally and inferiorly. The dorsal lingual artery is the major branch that arises from the lingual artery, usually below the hyoglossus muscle. At the level of the hyoid bone, it is located above it and medial to the hypoglossal nerve. Inferiorly located, with regard to the artery, lies the lingual vein that, in turn, accompanies the hypoglossal nerve.[15]

SPECIAL EQUIPMENT
Mouth Gags

In choosing an appropriate mouth gag or retractor for TORS surgery, the main consideration is whether the device provides adequate exposure to the anatomic structures without compromising the workspace necessary for the workings of the robotic arms and instruments. Two commonly used mouth gag systems are Davis Meyer (Karl Storz, USA) and Feyh-Kastenbauer-Weinstein-O'Malley (Gyrus ACMI, Germany). Each system includes multiple tongue blades of different lengths with integrated suction tubes for smoke evacuation. The ideal system is based on surgeon's preference.

Robot Instrumentation

The surgery is performed with the da Vinci Surgical system (Intuitive Surgical, Sunnyvale, CA, USA). The required robotic instrumentation includes the high-definition camera and the EndoWrist instruments (Intuitive Surgical, Sunnyvale, CA, USA).

High-definition camera
The binocular camera provides magnification of up to 10 times, which results in a 3D high-definition image that allows easy identification of vessels and nerves. It is available in 12-mm and 8-mm diameter scopes, both of which provide excellent optics while providing adequate working space in the mouth.

EndoWrist instruments
For TORS, two 5-mm articulated EndoWrist instrument arms are typically used. These instrument arms provide 180° of articulation and 540° of rotation, tremor filtration, amplitude scaling, and allow bimanual tissue manipulation in multiple planes. Typically, a grasper is placed in one arm and the spatula-tip monopolar cautery in the other for dissection and coagulation. Depending on surgeon preference, the monopolar cautery may be replaced with a compatible laser fiber. The grasping device is usually a 5-mm Maryland forceps.

Additional Equipment

Other TORS surgery equipment includes

1. Headlight
2. Suction cautery device
3. Yankauer suction device
4. Appropriate length forceps, hemostats, Metzenbaum scissors, and other basic soft tissue instruments.

PATIENT AND ROBOT POSITIONING
Operating Room Configuration

The patient cart should be centered with the surgeon console approximately 2.4 m away.[16] The surgeon console should be situated on the same side of the operating table as the assisting surgeon. This allows for easier communication between the assistant and the console surgeon. The anesthesia cart is placed at the foot of the bed (patient's head is turned 180° from anesthesia) and the assistant is seated at the head of the patient to provide suctioning and assistance with cauterization. The scrub nurse stands alongside the patient cart opposite to the robotic console.

Patient Positioning and Preparation

The patient is positioned supine, with or without a shoulder roll depending on the surgeon's preference and patient anatomy. Care must be taken to ensure that the patient's position on the bed allows proper positioning of the robotic base. In adjustable beds, this may not be an issue. However, with a nonadjustable base, the patient must be positioned with the head at the foot of the bed to allow room for the robotic base.

PROCEDURE
Anesthesia

During the preoperative and postoperative planning, a detailed discussion should occur with the anesthetic team because there is growing evidence that sleep apnea is a risk factor for anesthetic morbidity and mortality.[17] These patients are more likely to have comorbidities, including hypertension, esophageal and laryngopharyngeal reflux disease, coronary artery disease, and obesity. The importance of adequate postoperative analgesia that does not compromise respiratory function must be emphasized because these patients are at high risk of developing postoperative respiratory compromise from a combination of worsening sleep apnea, upper airway swelling, and narcotic analgesia. Monitoring these patients in a high dependency unit should be considered.

In addition, anatomic features present in these patients may lead to difficulty with intraoperative ventilation and intubation. Difficult-airway equipment, including a fiberoptic endoscope or GlideScope (Verathon Medical, Bothell, WA, USA), must be readily available. In Europe, it has been customary for patients undergoing a TORS tongue base resection to have a tracheostomy performed after intubation.[18] This is not routine in the United States and the surgery is typically performed via a nasotracheal tube.[19] Intravenous steroids are given intraoperatively and postoperatively to minimize lingual edema and nausea. If the airway is deemed at risk at the end of the procedure, the patient remains intubated until the upper airway swelling is minimized or a tracheotomy is performed.

Surgical Team

The primary surgeon
The primary surgeon is seated at the robotic console, which is typically in close proximity to the operating room table. The console affords a 3D view of the surgical field and allows manipulation of the two robotic arms and the camera.

The surgical assistant
The surgical assistant supports the primary surgeon by retracting tissues, creating a smoke-free environment, and suctioning blood to aid visualization. As needed, the assistant helps with adjusting the robotic arms and camera to prevent collisions, as well as facilitate hemostasis using suction diathermy or through the application of

vessel clips. There is an integrated microphone-loudspeaker system inbuilt in the robotic system that aids communication between the primary and assistant surgeon.

The surgical scrub

The surgical scrub aids in passing instruments and providing equipment as needed but may also provide assistance with suctioning. It is imperative that the surgical scrub is familiar with the TORS setup to aid in both decreasing setup and operative time.

The assistant surgeon and the surgical scrub can see a two-dimensional representation of the surgeon's view on the slave monitor, which is attached to the robot in the da Vinci S HD model and to the control tower–vision cart in the Si model.

Surgical Steps

Operative setup

The patient is positioned supine and the upper airway is anesthetized with topical lidocaine. As described in the literature, a sleep endoscopy is performed to assess the sites of obstruction.[20–22] The patient is then intubated with a nasotracheal tube and the operating table is turned 180° from the anesthesia cart. A stitch is placed in the anterior portion of the tongue to assist in retraction and positioning of the tongue. The mouth gag is placed to provide adequate exposure of the base of the tongue. At this point, the surgical bed is lowered to the lowest position possible. The robotic patient side cart is wheeled to the patient's head so that the base of the cart is approximately on a 30° angle with the base of the surgical bed. The robotic base may come from either the left or right side depending on the room setup.

The three robotic arms are positioned in a triangular format. The camera is placed in the center arm and the grasping instrument and cutting instrument are placed on the side arms depending on which side of the base of the tongue is addressed first. The instruments are inserted into the patient's mouth so that the apexes of the instruments meet in the operative area. Care must be taken to ensure that the instruments themselves do not collide and that their movement is not obstructed by intraoral structures.

Right-side lingual tonsillectomy

The base of the tongue is viewed using the 30° 12-mm camera, facing up. The Maryland 5-mm forceps are placed in the left arm and the spatula-tip cautery in the right arm. The incision begins in the midline and extends from the foramen caecum to the vallecula. This effectively splits the lingual tonsillar tissue in half; the deep extent of the incision is the junction between the lymphoid tissue and the underlying muscle.

The borders of the right lingual tonsil are identified and marked with cautery to outline the resection margins. This is comprised superiorly from the sulcus terminalis, laterally from the glossopharyngeal sulcus, and inferiorly to the glossoepiglottic sulcus.

The outlined tissue is then resected, with the deep plane being formed by the junction between the lymphoid tissue and underlying muscle. This is usually done in an en bloc fashion with minimal blood loss. The assistant facilitates this resection by using a suction or a retracting device for countertraction of the tissue. The inferior limit of the surgical bed is recognized by a bluish color of the vallecular mucosa. Several small vessel branches from the lingual artery are encountered and are controlled with electrocautery. Larger vessels are clipped as needed. Visualization of these vessels is improved by increasing the scope magnification.

Left-sided lingual tonsillectomy

The spatula-tip monopolar cautery is now placed in the left instrument arm and the grasping forceps in the right. The above steps are repeated.

Residual obstructive evaluation

Additional tissue is removed as needed to assure an adequate view of the airway. A minimal overall volume of 7 cc is recommended for fixing obstruction. It is usually safe to remove a layer of muscle less than or equal to 10 mm within the tongue base surgical site. Usually, an additional 5-mm thick strip of muscle may be safely removed in the tongue base within 5 mm of either side of the midline without encountering the hypoglossal nerves.

This additional midline muscle resection must be done carefully and under sufficiently high magnification. It is of paramount importance to use the midline of the tongue base as the point of reference to minimize the risk to the hypoglossal nerve, lingual artery, and lingual neural branches. Because of inherent anatomic variability, and tissue distortion from tongue retraction and mouth gag placement, precise localization of these structures is not possible.[23–25]

Supraglottoplasty

This optional step is performed at the same operative setting immediately after completion of the tongue base resection. Supraglottoplasty is designed to ameliorate the inward inspiratory collapse of floppy and/or redundant epiglottic, aryepiglottic, and/or arytenoid mucosa.[2,26,27]

The epiglottis is incised in the midline, following the medial glossoepiglottic fold. This split begins at the epiglottic tip and extends to approximately 5 mm above the vallecula. A sufficient amount of epiglottic height must be left to minimize the chance for aspiration.

The inferior extent of the midline epiglottic split is extended laterally on both sides. The plane of resection is above the pharyngoepiglottic folds to minimize the chance of aspiration and to avoid bleeding from branches of the superior laryngeal vessels. In addition to stabilizing this supraglottic tissue, the secondary intention is that healing in the vallecula and adjacent areas from this procedure results in anterior advancement of the epiglottis. Overly aggressive resection of epiglottic tissue must be avoided to prevent aspiration.

POSTOPERATIVE MANAGEMENT

The initial postoperative observation should be undertaken in a high-dependency unit given the potential for bleeding and/or airway edema after TORS tongue base surgery. Continuous pulse-oximetry is recommended. Postoperative intravenous steroids may help with nausea, airway edema, and pain from the inflammatory response. Consideration should be given to placement of a nasogastric feeding tube. Some centers routinely use a nasogastric tube for all TORS patients in the immediate postoperative period. This decision may be made according to the surgeon's preference and the patient's wishes.

As is the case with all such pharyngeal surgical defects, the risk of postoperative bleeding has a bimodal distribution, with one peak within hours of surgery and the second within 7 to 10 days of surgery. Patients must be advised of this risk and told to present to an emergency department immediately should any bleeding occur. This bleeding, as with routine posttonsillectomy hemorrhage, is treated conservatively or operatively, depending on severity.

Patients are followed closely after discharge. Diet is normalized as healing progresses and formal therapist-directed swallowing therapy is used as required. Postoperative polysomnography is performed once healing is complete, usually at least 3 to 6 months following surgery.

Table 1 Complications TORS for OSAHS (unpublished data from 75 consecutive patients)	
Operative Complications	**Percentage (%)**
Transient hypogeusia	18.3
Intraoperative or postoperative pharyngeal edema	3.16
Late self-limited bleeding	2.5
Teeth injury	0.0
Pharyngeal wall penetration	0.0
Intraoperative bleeding	0.0
Revision surgery	0.0
Death	0.0

COMPLICATIONS

The largest series of patients to undergo TORS for OSAHS has been performed by Vicini and colleagues.[15] The most common operative complications include hypogeusia, transient pharyngeal edema, and limited bleeding (**Table 1**). The pressure from the tongue blade attached to the mouth gag may cause temporary injury to the lingual nerve resulting in numbness that typically resolves in 1 to 4 weeks. Pharyngeal edema may also occur because of the pressure from the tongue blade and heat generated from the monopolar cautery. Both of these complications are directly related to the length of the operation and amount of time the patient is kept in suspension. Patients in suspension for less than 45 minutes are less likely to develop these complications.

Late self-limiting bleeding is uncommon and is reported in 2.5% of cases. More severe complications (teeth injury, pharyngeal wall penetration, intraoperative bleeding requiring open control of vessels, and death) have not been reported.

OUTCOME

The series reported by Vicini and colleagues (**Fig. 1**) showed an improvement from a mean preoperative AHI of 36.3 to a postoperative AHI of 16.4. Fifteen of the

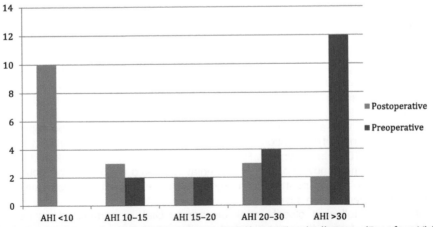

Fig. 1. Preoperative and postoperative AHI as reported by Vicini and colleagues. (*Data from* Vicini C, et al. Transoral robotic surgery of the tongue base in obstructive sleep Apnea-Hypopnea syndrome: anatomic considerations and clinical experience. Head Neck 2012;34(1):15–22.)

20 patients in this series had a postoperative AHI less than 20 and only two patients had an AHI greater than 30. Improvements were also seen in Epworth Sleepiness Scale, lowest oxygen saturation, and overall patient satisfaction. All improvements were found statistically significant.

SUMMARY

The role of surgery for the treatment of OSAHS is much debated[28] and currently lacks a comprehensive randomized evidence base mostly because of the heterogeneous nature of the disease itself and the range of surgical techniques used. Although many patients benefit from the use of the gold-standard therapy of CPAP, noncompliant patients require an alternative. Surgery, in suitable patients, offers this alternative. The application of TORS to the surgical treatment of OSAHS is still in its infancy; however, the results, so far, are promising. TORS for OSAHS allows the surgeon to address base-of-tongue obstruction with excellent visualization and a minimally invasive approach that is well tolerated by the patient. Currently, there are limited data to support its success; however, the evidence base is growing and it is hoped that TORS for OSAHS continues to show a positive benefit.

REFERENCES

1. Hobson JC, Robinson S, Antic NA, et al. What is "success" following surgery for obstructive sleep apnea? The effects of different polysomnographic scoring system. Laryngoscope 2012;122(8):1878–81.
2. Vicini C, Dallan I, Canzi P, et al. Transoral robotic tongue base resection in obstructive sleep apnea-hypopnea syndrome: a preliminary report. ORL J Otorhinolaryngol Relat Spec 2010;72(1):22–7.
3. Lin HS, Rowley JA, Badr MS, et al. Transoral robotic surgery for treatment of obstructive sleep apnea-hypopnea syndrome. Laryngoscope 2013;123(7): 1811–6.
4. Sher AE, Kenneth KB, Jay FB. The efficacy of surgical modifications of the upper airway in adults with obstructive sleep apnea syndrome. Sleep 1996;19:156–77.
5. Vicini F, Montevecchi F, Pang K, et al. Combined transoral robotic tongue base surgery and palate surgery in obstructive sleep apnea-hypopnea syndrome: expansion sphincter pharyngoplasty versus uvulopalatopharyngoplasty. Head Neck 2014;36(1):77–83.
6. Lee JM, Weinstein GS, O'Malley BW, et al. Transoral robot-assisted lingual tonsillectomy and uvulopalatopharyngoplasty for obstructive sleep apnea. Ann Otol Rhinol Laryngol 2012;121(10):635–9.
7. Weaver EM. Judging sleep apnea surgery. Sleep Med Rev 2010;14:283–5.
8. Yaggi HK, Concato J, Kernan WN, et al. Obstructive sleep apnea as a risk factor for stroke and death. N Engl J Med 2005;353:2034–41.
9. Peker Y, Hedner J, Norum J, et al. Increased incidence of cardiovascular disease in middle-aged men with obstructive sleep apnea: a 7-year follow-up. Am J Respir Crit Care Med 2002;166(2):159–65.
10. Parati G, Lombardi C, Narkiewicz K. Sleep apnea: epidemiology, pathophysiology, and relation to cardiovascular risk. Am J Physiol Regul Integr Comp Physiol 2007;293:R1671–83.
11. Greenburg DL, Lettieri CJ, Eliasson AH. Effects of surgical weight loss on measures of obstructive sleep apnea: a meta-analysis. Am J Med 2009;122:535–42.
12. Ravesloot MJL, de Vries N. Reliable calculation of the efficacy of non-surgical and surgical treatment of obstructive sleep apnea. Sleep 2011;34(1):105–10.

13. Vicini C, Montevecchi F, Magnuson JS. Robotic surgery for obstructive sleep apnea. Curr Otorhinolaryngol Rep 2013;1:130–6.
14. Haraldsson PO, Carenfelt C, Lysdahl M, et al. Does uvulopalatopharyngoplasty inhibit automobile accidents? Laryngoscope 1995;105:657–61.
15. Vicini C, Dallan I, Canzi P, et al. Transoral robotic surgery of the tongue base in obstructive sleep Apnea-Hypopnea syndrome: anatomic considerations and clinical experience. Head Neck 2012;34(1):15–22.
16. White HN, Frederick J, Zimmerman T, et al. Learning curve for transoral robotic surgery: a 4-year analysis. JAMA 2013;139(6):564–7.
17. Michelson SA. Preoperative and postoperative management of obstructive sleep apnea patients. Otolaryngol Clin North Am 2007;40:877–89.
18. Campanini A, De Vito A, Frassineti S, et al. Temporary tracheotomy in the surgical treatment of obstructive sleep apnea syndrome: personal experience. Acta Otorhinolaryngol Ital 2003;23(6):474–8.
19. Friedman M, Hamilton C, Samuelson CG, et al. Transoral robotic glossectomy for the treatment of obstructive sleep apnea-hypopnea syndrome. Otolaryngol Head Neck Surg 2012;146(5):854–62.
20. Hohenhorst W, Ravesloot MJ, Kezirian EJ, et al. Drug-induced sleep endoscopy in adults with sleep-disordered breathing: technique and the vote classification system. Operative Techniques in Otolaryngology 2012;23(1):11–8.
21. Kezirian EJ. Nonresponders to pharyngeal surgery for obstructive sleep apnea: insights from drug-induced sleep endoscopy. Laryngoscope 2011;121:1320–6.
22. Rabelo FA, Braga A, Kupper DS, et al. Propofol-induced sleep: polysomnographic evaluation of patients with obstructive sleep apnea and controls. JAMA 2010;142(2):218–24.
23. Vicini C, Montevecchi F, Dallan I, et al. Transoral robotic geniohyoidpexy as an additional step of transoral robotic tongue base reduction and supraglottoplasty: feasibility in a cadaver model. ORL J Otorhinolaryngol Relat Spec 2011;73(3): 147–50.
24. Sequert C, Lestang P, Baglin AC, et al. Hypoglossal nerve in its intralingual trajectory: anatomy and clinical implications. Ann Otolaryngol Chir Cervicofac 1999; 116(4):207–17.
25. Lauretano AM, Li KK, Caradonna DS, et al. Anatomic location of the tongue base neurovascular bundle. Laryngoscope 1997;107(8):1057–9.
26. Vicini C, Montevecchi F, Tenti G, et al. Transoral robotic surgery: tongue base reduction and supraglottoplasty for obstructive sleep apnea. Operative Technique in Otolaryngology 2012;23(1):45–7.
27. Golz A, Goldenberg D, Westerman ST, et al. Laser partial epiglottidectomy as a treatment for obstructive sleep apnea and laryngomalacia. Ann Otol Rhinol Laryngol 2000;109(12):1140–5.
28. MacKay SG, Weaver EM. Surgery for obstructive sleep apnoea. Med J Aust 2013;199(7):450–1.

Transoral Robotic Surgery (TORS) for Benign Pharyngeal Lesions

Jason Y.K. Chan, MBBS, Jeremy D. Richmon, MD*

KEYWORDS

- Nasopharynx • Oropharynx • Hypopharynx • Transoral robotic surgery • TORS
- Benign • Robot • Minimally invasive

KEY POINTS

- TORS for benign pharyngeal lesions follows similar operative set-up and technique as for malignant lesions, often with less destruction of normal tissue.
- Placement of tracheotomy and gastrostomy tube are not expected.
- One much always consider the location of the dorsal lingual artery and carotid artery.
- Placement of a nasogastric feeding tube is recommended if a palatal split approach is utilized.

INTRODUCTION

The first robotic system, known as the Automated Endoscopic System for Optimal Positioning, was approved by the Food and Drug Administration (FDA) in 1993. It provided a robotically controlled arm to manipulate an endoscope for laparoscopic surgery. This system subsequently evolved to the development of the da Vinci Surgical System (Intuitive Surgical, Inc, Sunnyvale, CA, USA), which was FDA approved for abdominal laparoscopic surgery in 2000 and more recently for transoral otolaryngology surgical procedures restricted to T1 and T2 benign and malignant lesions in 2009.

The da Vinci robot consists of several key components: the surgeon console, the patient-side cart, the vision system, and the endowrist instruments. The surgeon console provides a 3-dimensional (3D), high-definition image of the operative field and the master controls for the robotic arms and video endoscope. It is positioned at a distance from the patient. The patient-side cart is positioned next to the patient and includes 3 or 4 robotic arms delivering the surgical instruments and video endoscope.

Conflict of Interest: J.D. Richmon, MD is a consultant for Intuitive Surgical, Inc.
Department of Otolaryngology–Head and Neck Surgery, Johns Hopkins Hospital, Baltimore, MD 21287, USA
* Corresponding author. Department of Otolaryngology–Head and Neck Surgery, JHOC 6th Floor, 601 North Caroline Street, Baltimore, MD 21287.
E-mail address: Jrichmo7@jhmi.edu

This robot is a master-slave system and surgeon input is required for all robotic movement. The vision system includes a 3D high-definition 0° or 30° endoscope coupled to an image-processing tower and monitor for the operating room staff and assisting surgeon. The endowrist effector arms are articulating wristed instruments with 7 degrees of freedom in both 8-mm and 5-mm sizes. The operative table is typically rotated so the patient's head is opposite from the anesthesia cart. The patient is appropriately relaxed to allow for the placement of a mouth gag and suspension. Dental protection is recommended. Three of the robotic arms (scope in the center flanked by right and left 5-mm effector arms) are advanced through the mouth. A 0° or 30° scope can be used for tonsil resections and a 30° scope affords optimal visualization of the tongue base and hypopharynx. The assisting surgeon sits at the head of the bed and uses an instrument (typically a suction, cautery, retractor, or clip device) in each hand. This configuration allows for 2 surgeons and 4 instruments working at the same time in the pharynx.

Transoral robotic surgery (TORS) provides the surgeon with a 3D, high-definition view of the operative field from the perspective of being inside the mouth of the patient. The maneuverable scope affords a wide field of vision. The wristed instruments with tremor-filtration, motion-scaling, and 7 degrees of freedom provide precise bimanual tissue manipulation in areas heretofore inaccessible through the mouth, allowing for en-bloc excision and complete visualization of large tumors through the mouth and obviating an external approach and cervical scar. A frequently cited limitation of the robot is the lack of haptic feedback, which many experts feel is compensated for by the superior 3D vision. For the purpose of this article, the use of TORS is examined in the treatment of benign lesions of the pharynx, subdivided into the nasopharynx, oropharynx, and hypopharynx.

PREOPERATIVE IMAGING

Preoperative planning primarily involves using computed tomography (CT) and magnetic resonance imaging (MRI). CT with intravenous contrast provides information on the nasopharynx regarding the status of the skull base, clivus, and pterygoid plates and the relationship of the lesion to the internal carotid artery. In the oropharynx it provides information regarding the location, extent, and vascularity of the lesion in question. In the hypopharynx, CT imaging defines the status of the arytenoids, thyroid cartilage, and proximity to the common carotid artery. MRI provides more soft tissue detail and depth information of the lesions in the nasopharynx, oropharynx, and hypopharynx. In addition, the soft tissue characteristics may assist in the differentiation of a malignant from a benign lesion. Furthermore, CT or MRI may be used in cases whereby navigation is desired, such as described in a combined endoscopic and TORS approach to lesions in the nasopharynx.[1]

NASOPHARYNGEAL LESIONS
Patient Setup

The patient is placed supine on the operative table and intubated orally. A small endotracheal tube taped to the midline or off to the side affords the most room to work through the mouth. Dental protection with a thermoplastic splint is recommended. The head is kept midline with the neck extended. Muscle relaxation is necessary. A Crowe-Davis or Dingman retractors are most frequently used to open the mouth widely. It is the authors' practice to administer antibiotics covering mixed pharyngeal flora as well as steroids intraoperatively, which is thought to reduce edema, postoperative pain, nausea, and vomiting. As most procedures last less than 2 hours, there is no need for placement of a urinary catheter unless additional procedures are performed or medical condition warrants.

The table is rotated 180° from anesthesia to maximize exposure to the patient's head. The robot is docked from either the left or the right side at a 30° angle to the bed. The assistant sits at the head of the bed with a clear view into the mouth as well as to the video cart monitor, which shows the endoscopic view.

Surgical Technique

Nasopharyngeal dissection was initially described by Ozer and Waltonen,[2] in which a Dingman retractor was used for transoral exposure. All 4 robotic arms were placed through the mouth with a 30° scope facing superiorly. The soft palate was incised lateral to midline and separated from the attachments to the hard palate and pharyngeal wall and the opposite soft palate and uvula were retracted with the fourth robot arm, allowing for adequate exposure of the nasopharynx. Similar to the above technique, Wei and Ho[3] described adequate visualization and access to the nasopharynx between the 2 posterior crura of the eustachian tubes with a 0° camera. This technique uses a lateral palatal flap approach whereby an incision is carried from the incisive foramen to the greater palatine foramen contralateral to the tumor (**Fig. 1**). The incision is carried onto the soft palate toward the superior pole of the tonsil 1 cm medial to the gingiva, which affords better access to the lateral nasopharynx and parapharyngeal space.[4] Care must be taken not to injure the contralateral greater palatine vessels because they are the dependent supply of the palatal flap.

Within the nasopharynx, TORS has been described in the treatment of small recurrent nasopharyngeal carcinomas that are not contiguous with the internal carotid artery.[1,4] Benign lesions are relatively rare in the nasopharynx and may include papillomas, teratomas, pedunculated fibromas, fibromyxomatous polyps, and Tornwaldt cysts. Admittedly, most of these lesions are accessible through standard transnasal endoscopic sinus surgery techniques. Current instrumentation of the da Vinci robot does not allow for sufficient articulation and camera flexibility to access the entire nasopharynx without

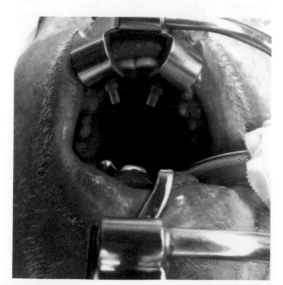

Fig. 1. A crow-davis mouth gag has been placed to expose the hard and soft palate. An incision has been marked for a lateral palatal approach to the nasopharynx.

a palatal split and/or extended approach (e.g. transfacial or transcervical) therefore this technique should be reserved for significantly larger tumors with an inferior extent not completely accessible via sinus endoscopy.

OROPHARYNGEAL LESIONS
Patient Setup

Patient setup and positioning are similar to that described above for tonsillar and posterior pharyngeal wall lesions. A 0° scope is usually adequate for these areas. However, for base of tongue lesions. A 2-0 silk suture is placed in the posterior tongue and pulled anteriorly for mouth gag placement. While extracting the tongue, a Feyh-Kastenbauer (FK) retractor with the appropriate tongue blade is inserted and suspended on a Louis arm stand. Adequate tension on the silk suture is mandatory to pull the base of tongue anteriorly and often to the contralateral side to allow visualization and access to the oropharynx. If inadequate exposure is obtained initially, the various FK retractor tongue blades should be tried to obtain a better view. A 30 degree scope may be helpful to visualize down into the vallecula. A spatula tip Bovie cautery is placed ipsilateral to the lesion and a Maryland dissector is placed in the contralateral arm allowing the lesion to be pulled to the contralateral side as dissection proceeds with the Bovie cautery, as shown in **Fig. 2**.

Surgical Technique

The first application of the da Vinci robot in the head and neck, as described by McLeod and Melder in 2005,[5] was for a vallecular cyst, which was marsupialized

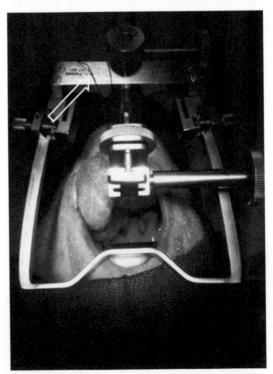

Fig. 2. Feyh-Kastenbauer (FK) retractor in place with a suture (*arrow*) used to pull the tongue anteriorly and to the contralateral side of the lesion to maximize exposure.

through a suspended slotted laryngoscope. There have also been reports of 2 lingual thyroid glands and one lingual thyroglossal duct cyst excised robotically (**Table 1**).[6–8] The extent of the resection is dictated by the size of the lesion. For base of tongue lesions a mucosal cut is made anterior to the lesion followed by medial and lateral cuts with cautery. Then a shelf is created through the anterior mucosal incision cutting deep in the direction of the vallecula, taking care to remain pericapsular. This part can be challenging in that identification of the capsule may not be obvious until after it is violated. Therefore, usually a small cuff of normal tissue is taken around the lesion, even if it is benign, to prevent inadvertent incomplete resections. The removal of a cuff of normal tissue is especially important for pleomorphic adenomas where care must be taken to carry this shelf anteriorly into the deep tongue musculature to avoid capsular violation and potential spillage. The dorsal lingual artery may be encountered laterally and, if traced proximal, will lead to the lingual artery. If violated, this vessel can bleed profusely and therefore must be controlled with a hemoclip and/or cautery. Another consideration is the hypoglossal nerve that is found anterolateral to the dorsal lingual artery; this is encountered during lateral dissection, and the distal portion of the nerve may be resected as dictated by the extent of the tumor.[9,10] The authors do not routinely perform a tracheotomy. If there is concern of significant airway compromise at the end of the surgery, We recommend leaving the patient intubated overnight until safe extubation is possible. Placing a thin-bore feeding tube intraoperatively as a precautionary measure for dysphagia is recommended.

HYPOPHARYNGEAL LESIONS
Patient Setup

The approach to the hypopharynx is similar to that of the base of the tongue. The patient is placed in the Boyce position and a tooth guard is placed over the upper dentition, and the FK retractor is then used with a tongue spade blade that allows an adequate surgical view and access space to the hypopharynx.[11,12]

Surgical Technique

Park and colleagues[11] describe a total pyriform sinus resection that can be used as a basis for resection of primary malignant lesions. For benign lesions a variation of this technique is used such that there is less extensive resection while still removing the entire lesion. The most challenging aspect of resecting lesions in the hypopharynx is gaining exposure to the hypopharynx and being able to reach and manipulate the lesion with the robotic arms. This aspect is not possible in many patients with current robotic technology. The parallel conformation of the instruments causes frequent

Table 1
List of cases of benign lesions of the oropharynx

Study	Pathology	Diet	LOS (d)	Complications	Notes
McLeod & Melder,[5] 2005	Vallecular cyst	POD 0	0	None	Marsupialization of cyst
May et al,[8] 2011	Lingual thyroid	N/A	3	None	None
Kimple et al,[6] 2012	Lingual TDC	POD 1	1	None	None
Dallan et al,[7] 2013	Lingual thyroid	POD 1	13	None	Required tracheostomy

Abbreviations: LOS, length of stay; POD, postoperative day; TDC, thyroglossal duct cyst.
Data from Refs.[5–8]

collisions of the external arms, which may preclude safe utilization of the da Vinci in patients with difficulty in neck extension, a small mandibular arch, reduced mouth opening, or a significantly anterior airway. Larger patients with a wide mouth opening are more favorable, especially if edentulous. Operating in the narrow confines of the hypopharynx can be disorienting and it is helpful to maintain a clear landmark (ie, arytenoid, vocal cord, epiglottis) within the endoscopic view to maintain orientation. Patients with benign hypopharyngeal lesions, such as lipoma, fibroma, leiomyoma, and granular cell tumors, can often avoid a tracheotomy following robotic resection. Of course, the degree of airway edema and swallow dysfunction is proportional to the size of resection and amount of normal tissue removed.

POSTOPERATIVE MANAGEMENT
Nasopharynx

For benign lesions there should be no need to incise through the pharyngobasilar fascia exposing the clivus, and wounds should be allowed to heal by secondary intention. However, if there is bone exposed and coverage is needed, free mucosal grafts or a nasoseptal flap may be used with temporary packing for 4 to 5 days to allow for healing before removal.[3,4] Patients with palatal incisions should also be temporarily fed through a nasal feeding tube to allow for healing.

Oropharynx and Hypopharynx

An oral diet can usually be initiated on postoperative day 1. This can be safely accomplished after passing a bedside swallow examination performed by a speech language pathologist or experienced physician. The feeding tube is removed and a liquid diet is begun with directions to advance as tolerated on discharge home. Alternatively, if there is evidence of aspiration, tube feeds can be initiated and swallow function can be reassessed at a later date. Steroids are given intravenously for 24 hours to help with surgical site edema, pain, and nausea. Longer steroid administration may increase the likelihood of oropharyngeal candidiasis.

SUMMARY

Although TORS has a well-established role in the treatment of malignant lesions of the nasopharynx, oropharynx, and hypopharynx, there exist relatively few reports on the treatment of benign lesions in these same areas. Nonetheless, room setup, patient positioning, robotic technique, and perioperative care are essentially identical to that for malignant lesions, with the difference in the extent of resection. Therefore, it can be extrapolated that the promising functional outcomes of TORS in the treatment of malignant lesions should be equivalent, if not better, for benign lesions. TORS offers a superb, minimally invasive technique to remove lesions of the pharynx.

REFERENCES

1. Yin Tsang RK, Ho WK, Wei WI. Combined transnasal endoscopic and transoral robotic resection of recurrent nasopharyngeal carcinoma. Head Neck 2012; 34(8):1190–3.
2. Ozer E, Waltonen J. Transoral robotic nasopharyngectomy: a novel approach for nasopharyngeal lesions. Laryngoscope 2008;118(9):1613–6.
3. Wei WI, Ho WK. Transoral robotic resection of recurrent nasopharyngeal carcinoma. Laryngoscope 2010;120(10):2011–4.

4. Tsang RK, Mohr C. Lateral palatal flap approach to the nasopharynx and para-pharyngeal space for transoral robotic surgery: a cadaveric study. J Robot Surg 2013;7(2):119–23.
5. McLeod IK, Melder PC. Da Vinci robot-assisted excision of a vallecular cyst: a case report. Ear Nose Throat J 2005;84(3):170–2.
6. Kimple AJ, Eliades SJ, Richmon JD. Transoral robotic resection of a lingual thy-roglossal duct cyst. J Robot Surg 2012;6(4):367–9.
7. Dallan I, Montevecchi F, Seccia V, et al. Transoral robotic resection of an ectopic tongue-base thyroid gland. J Robot Surg 2013;7(1):83–6.
8. May JT IV, Newman JG, Padhya TA. Transoral robotic-assisted excision of a lingual thyroid gland. J Robot Surg 2011;5(3):217–20.
9. Moore EJ, Janus J, Kasperbauer J. Transoral robotic surgery of the oropharynx: clinical and anatomic considerations. Clin Anat 2012;25(1):135–41.
10. Moore EJ, Olsen KD, Kasperbauer JL. Transoral robotic surgery for oropharyn-geal squamous cell carcinoma: a prospective study of feasibility and functional outcomes. Laryngoscope 2009;119(11):2156–64.
11. Park YM, Kim WS, Byeon HK, et al. Feasibility of transoral robotic hypopharyng-ectomy for early-stage hypopharyngeal carcinoma. Oral Oncol 2010;46(8):597–602.
12. Park YM, Lee WJ, Lee JG, et al. Transoral robotic surgery (TORS) in laryngeal and hypopharyngeal cancer. J Laparoendosc Adv Surg Tech A 2009;19(3):361–8.

Robotic Surgery of the Skull Base

Michael E. Kupferman, MD*, Ehab Hanna, MD

KEYWORDS

- Robotics • Surgery • Skull base • Pituitary • Reconstruction

KEY POINTS

- Although still in the developmental stages, robotic applications to skull base surgery are forthcoming.
- Transantral robotic surgery provides stereoscopic endoscopic access to the anterior skull base and pituitary fossa, and allows 2-handed endoscopic manipulation and reconstruction.
- Traditional suture and reconstructive techniques can be implemented in this confined surgical site with the use of robotic technology.
- Future development and refinement of endonasal robotic instrumentation is critical before applying these techniques in the clinical setting.

INTRODUCTION

In the past several years, transnasal endoscopic approaches have been increasingly used for surgical access and treatment of neoplastic and benign lesions of the anterior and central skull base. Endoscopic surgery is used with increasing frequency for surgical resection of tumors of the sinonasal tract, such as inverted papilloma, angiofibroma, osteoma, and other benign fibro-osseous lesions, and in selected patients with malignant sinonasal tumors.[1–5] Endoscopic approaches are also becoming popular for transsphenoidal access to the sella turcica, and are considered by many centers to be the preferred surgical approach for treatment of pituitary adenomas.[6–9] More recently, there has been an emerging trend to expand the use of transnasal endoscopic approaches in the surgical treatment of suprasellar, petroclival, infratemporal, and other intracranial skull base tumors.[10–14]

The increasing popularity of these endoscopic skull base approaches may be attributed to a larger trend toward more minimally invasive techniques across all surgical

Disclosures: None.
Department of Head and Neck Surgery, MD Anderson Cancer Center, 1515 Holcombe Boulevard, Houston, TX 77030, USA
* Corresponding author. Department of Head and Neck Surgery, MD Anderson Cancer Center, 1400 Pressler Street, Unit 1445, Houston, TX 77030.
E-mail address: mekupfer@mdanderson.org

disciplines. The main advantage of transnasal endoscopic skull base approaches is providing more direct access to the anterior and central skull base while avoiding craniofacial incisions and extensive bone removal, which are commonly used in open surgical approaches. Also, the wider angle of vision and angled lenses increase the range of the endoscopic visual surgical field compared with the line-of-sight visual field gained by surgical loupes or microscopes.

One major disadvantage of transnasal endoscopic approaches is the inability to provide watertight dural closure and reconstruction, which limits its safety and widespread adoption in surgery for intradural skull base tumors. Current techniques of endoscopic skull base reconstruction, such as tissue grafts, mucosal flaps, and tissue sealants, provide adequate reconstruction of limited skull base defects, such as a posttraumatic cerebrospinal fluid leak.[15,16] However, for larger dural defects, these endoscopic techniques have higher cerebrospinal fluid leak rates compared with traditional reconstructive techniques used in open surgery, such as the vascularized pericranial flap.[10]

Although the application of robotic technology to surgery has rapidly expanded over the last 5 years, little-studied but fertile area for application of surgical robotics in the head and neck is minimally invasive skull base surgery. The advantages that these novel systems offer include the ability to perform bimanual surgery in confined cavities with instrumentation that exceeds the capabilities of the human hand, and providing the surgeon with a three-dimensional (3D) view of the surgical field. Significant advances in surgical robotics have been made,[17] although a role for robot-based applications in skull base surgery has not been completely defined.

TECHNIQUES
Approach to the Anterior Cranial Fossa

The feasibility of using the surgical robot to access the anterior and central skull base has been shown in a cadaver model.[18] Caldwell-Luc incisions and wide anterior maxillary antrostomies followed by wide middle meatal antrostomies are the entry points for the surgical arms (**Fig. 1**A). Sufficient access can be obtained without compromising the infraorbital nerves (see **Fig. 1**B), and a posterior septectomy provides a common bilateral surgical field. The robotic endoscope is then placed into the patient's nare and the right and left surgical arms are introduced through the respective maxillary sinuses (see **Fig. 1**C). Anterior and posterior ethmoidectomies are performed, and sphenoidotomies provide exposure to the planum sphenoidale, sella turcica, and parasellar regions (**Fig. 2**). With current technology, this is best performed using traditional transnasal endoscopic techniques before docking the robotic patient cart. In addition, current robotic instrumentation does not include a drill, although prototypes are under preclinical investigation. Therefore, removal of the anterior skull base bone is

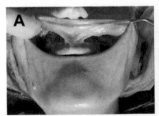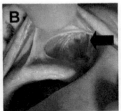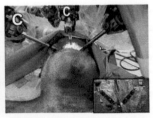

Fig. 1. (*A*) Sublabial incisions with bilateral exposure of the face of the maxilla. (*B*) Identification and preservation of the infraorbital nerve (*arrow*). (*C*) Docking of the camera (C) and the robotic arms via maxillary antrotomies.

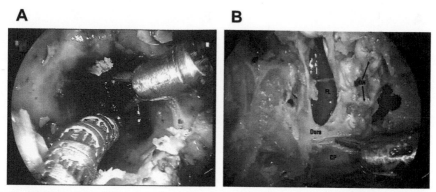

Fig. 2. (*A*) Dissection of the posterior wall of the sphenoid sinus. (*B*) The cribriform plate (CP) is removed bilaterally, and the cut edges of the olfactory nerves (ON) are shown; the dura is incised or resected to expose the inferior surface of the frontal lobes (FL) intracranially.

likewise best performed without robotic assistance. Access to the anterior cranial fossa is provided by sharp dissection of the anterior skull base and incision of the dura (**Fig. 3**A, B). The dual robotic arms can be used for primary repair of the dura.[19] This approach provides excellent access to the anterior and central skull base, including the cribriform plate, fovea ethmoidalis, medial orbits, planum sphenoidale, nasopharynx, pterygopalatine fossa, and clivus. The most significant advantage of this approach is the ability to perform 2-handed tremor-free endoscopic closure of dural defects. To date, this approach remains investigational.

Approach to the Pituitary Fossa

Although the transnasal endoscopic approach to the pituitary fossa has become a widely used technique for surgical resection,[20,21] robotic surgery in this anatomic location may provide unique advantages compared with the 4-handed technique. The feasibility of a robotic approach to the pituitary fossa has been described by the authors, and remains investigational.[22]

Similar to the approach to the anterior cranial fossa, access involves creating bilateral maxillary antrostomies and docking the robotic arms and camera, as described earlier. An anterior sphenoidotomy is then performed, and the sellar floor is removed to expose the dura of the pituitary fossa (**Fig. 4**). The dura is opened sharply with the robotic scissors to allow for exploration of the pituitary gland (**Fig. 5**A). Blunt and sharp

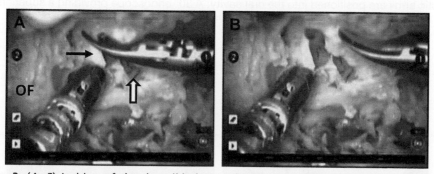

Fig. 3. (*A, B*) Incision of the dura (*black arrow*) with the robotic instrumentation after complete exposure of medial orbital walls and sphenoid sinus. The frontal lobe is visible (*white arrow*). OF, orbital fat.

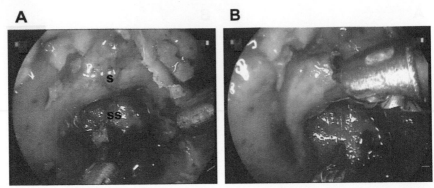

Fig. 4. (*A*) Exposure of the anterior face of the sella. (*B*) Entry into the pituitary fossa. S, sella; SS, sphenoid sinus.

dissection may be then performed to excise the pituitary gland after the optic chiasm and hypothalamus are exposed (see **Fig. 5**B). Dissection of the lateral wall of the sphenoid sinus may also be performed with high-speed drills and fine rongeurs to access the cavernous sinus. Using this technique, access to the central skull base, including the planum sphenoidale, the pituitary gland, cavernous carotid, mammillary bodies, and optic chiasm can be achieved.

A transcervical approach to the skull base in canine and cadaver models has previously been described. Access to the sphenoid, clivus, sella, and suprasellar anterior fossa can be obtained by placing a 30° robotic endoscope transorally and placing the right and left robotic arms through the lateral pharyngeal walls via a transcervical technique, posterior to the submandibular gland.[23]

Approach to the Nasopharynx

Robotic surgery of the nasopharynx is perhaps the only anatomic site of the skull base that is amenable to surgical dissection with current iterations of surgical robotics. The feasibility of robotic resection of nasopharyngeal lesions in a cadaver was first described in 2008,[24] and subsequent case reports of surgical management of nasopharyngeal cancers have been published in the literature.[25]

A Dingmann retractor is used to expose the oral cavity, and the soft palate is divided under direct visualization; lateral retraction of the divided palate is achieved with Vicryl suture (**Fig. 6**A). The da Vinci robot is then docked at the head of the bed, and the robotic arms are positioned into the oral cavity. A 30° endoscope providing a superiorly

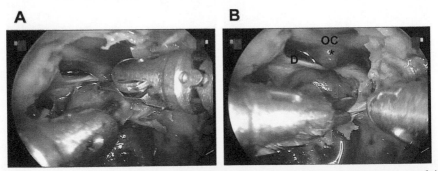

Fig. 5. (*A*) Resection of the pituitary gland. (*B*) Transected pituitary stalk and exposure of the optic chiasm. Asterisk, pituitary stalk; D, diaphragma sellae; OC, optic chiasm.

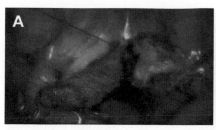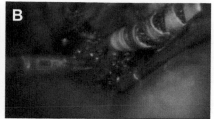

Fig. 6. (*A*) Exposure of the nasopharynx is achieved with a palatal split incision. (*B*) Incisions in the superior and inferior aspects of the nasopharynx commence the posterior dissection.

oriented view of the oropharynx and nasopharynx is typically used. Using the Maryland forceps and the spatula cautery, the nasopharynx soft tissue may then be progressively degloved (see **Fig. 6**B) between the carotid arteries and eustachian tubes laterally and the skull base and prevertebral musculature posteriorly. Once the tumor is resected, the palate is closed in 3 layers with absorbable suture. The advantage of this technique is that it allows en-bloc excision of nasopharyngeal lesions, and may offer the advantage of decreased morbidity compared with either reirradiation or open surgical approaches for recurrent nasopharyngeal carcinoma. Further study is necessary to delineate the optimal surgical indications.

Approach to the Infratemporal Fossa

Both preclinical studies and case reports addressing the infratemporal fossa and parapharyngeal space via robotic approaches have been described.[26,27] Dissection is performed through the lateral pharyngeal wall to access the parapharyngeal space. Using the 30° endoscope superiorly, the parapharyngeal space can be carefully explored to identify the neurovascular contents: jugular vein, internal carotid, and cranial nerves IX, X, XI, and XII. To gain exposure superiorly and laterally (to the infratemporal fossa), the styloid musculature can be resected and pterygoid muscles partially released. This approach may be best suited for well-circumscribed benign lesions.

Skull Base Reconstruction

Perhaps the most significant limitation of current transnasal endoscopic techniques is the inability to reconstruct dural defects with a sutured watertight dural closure. Options for repair of the skull base include free mucosal grafts, fascia lata grafts, pedicled mucosal grafts, and biological materials.[15,16,28–30] Although each has advantages and disadvantages, only the pedicled mucoperiosteal grafts are vascularized,[31] a necessary component of any reconstruction in patients undergoing postoperative irradiation, or in previously irradiated patients. One of the major drawbacks of the endoscopic approach is the inability to perform a suture-based reconstruction of the dura using currently available technology, an approach that is easily undertaken with a pericranial flap through the transcranial approach. We previously reported the feasibility of an endonasal robotic surgical dural reconstruction to address this problem in skull base surgery.

Repair of the skull base defect can be performed robotically with 2 distinct techniques. First, repair of the dura may be primarily reconstructed with both continuous and interrupted suture techniques (**Fig. 7**A). In addition, harvested sinonasal mucoperiosteal graft can be sutured into dural defects with both running and interrupted suture techniques (see **Fig. 7**B). Although these techniques have been shown in cadaver models, their application in human use has yet to be realized.

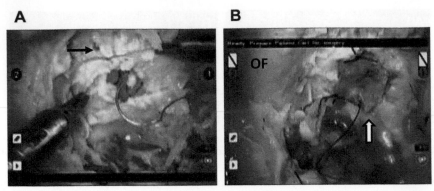

Fig. 7. (A) Primary repair of a dural defect (*black arrow*) with polyglactin suture (Ethicon). (B) Repair of a large dural defect with a mucosal graft (*white arrow*).

A balanced analysis of the place of robotic surgery on the spectrum of surgical modalities suggests that robot-assisted skull base surgery offers unique advantages that are lacking in either microscopic or transnasal endoscopic techniques. These advantages can be divided into 4 major areas: optical, ergonomic, dissection, and reconstructive. The following is a discussion of how endoscopic robotic surgery can overcome some of the limitations of these other techniques, and of the limitations of robotic surgery.

Optical limitations
The two-dimensional visualization provided by single-channel optical systems in current endoscopes lacks the depth perception of 3D vision provided by the binocular optical systems used in standard microsurgery. During endoscopic surgery, depth perception relies more on tactile than on visual cues. Visual depth perception is particularly important when operating on critical intracranial neurovascular structures, especially when working in a deep and limited space. The 5-mm robotic endoscope has a dual-channel optical system coupled with a dual charge-coupled device, which allows 3D visualization of the surgical field at the surgeon's console. This binocular endoscope allows the surgeon to have the combined benefit of a wider angle of vision and the depth perception of 3D visualization.

Ergonomic limitations
Current endoscopic techniques have several ergonomic limitations. Bimanual surgery is only feasible if the endoscope is held by an assistant or a mechanical holder. A surgical assistant is preferred because of the constant need to adjust the position (depth and angle) of the endoscope during endoscopic surgery, which not only limits the direct control of the endoscope by the primary surgeon but also requires the assistance of an experienced endoscopic surgeon who can seamlessly follow the primary surgeon in every step of the operation.

Also, both surgeons have to work within the confined space provided by the nostrils, which in some cases limits ergonomic freedom. In addition, as the surgical field gets deeper, longer instruments are needed and, with lack of proper arm support, precision may be limited by fine tremor, especially when using fine instrumentation for delicate dissection of critical neurovascular structures. The robotic system has 4 arms, all of which are controlled by the primary surgeon sitting at the console. One arm, the camera port, holds the endoscope; 2 arms hold right-hand and left-hand instruments; and a fourth, spare arm may be dedicated for retraction or a third instrument. This arrangement allows the primary surgeon simultaneous direct control of the endoscope and the instrumentation, an advantage that is not feasible with nonrobotic endoscopic techniques. Another advantage of the EndoWrist technology used in the da Vinci robotic instrumentation is its ability to provide movement at the instrument tip with 7° of freedom and 90° of articulation and motion scaling. This ability allows the surgeon, who sits comfortably at the console with an adjustable arm, support to perform precise tremor-free movement in a deep and confined space, with working angles that are usually not achievable with nonrobotic instruments.

Dissection limitations

In its current iteration, the da Vinci robotic system is designed exclusively for soft tissue surgery, whereas the paranasal sinuses and skull base are bony anatomic structures. Access to tumors in these domains requires bone-cutting instrumentation, including rongeurs, osteotomes, and drills. The exquisitely tuned internal pulley system within the robotic arms is not engineered for the stress forces that bony dissection requires. In our experience, use of the robotic dissecting instruments led to rapid deterioration in the functionality and life-span of the equipment. Further optimization of the robotic arms is required before skull base surgery can be performed effectively with the novel technology.

Reconstructive limitations

The most significant limitation of current transnasal endoscopic techniques is the inability to suture and provide watertight dural closure or reconstruction of dural defects. Endoscopic repair of dural defects relies on nonvascularized fat, mucosal or allogeneic grafts, or vascularized septal or nasal rotational mucosal flaps. These reconstructions are then covered with fibrin sealants and supported by either absorbable or nonabsorbable packing. Although these methods may provide adequate reconstruction of minor dural tears or defects, their ability to provide safe and reliable reconstruction of larger dural defects remains to be seen. Preliminary results suggest that these methods have a higher cerebrospinal fluid leak rate compared with the more standard dural reconstruction using pedicled (axial) flaps, such as the pericranial flap or microvascular free flaps. Adequate and reliable dural reconstruction is critical in minimizing the morbidity of skull base resections, particularly in patients who have received or are to undergo high-dose radiation therapy. As described earlier, robot-assisted surgery allows successful and precise endoscopic suturing of the dura, which may drastically affect the usefulness and safety of endoscopic surgery of intracranial intradural lesions of the skull base.

SUMMARY

Although still in the developmental stages, robotic applications to skull base surgery are forthcoming. Transantral robotic surgery provides stereoscopic endoscopic access to the anterior skull base and pituitary fossa, and allows 2-handed endoscopic manipulation and reconstruction. Traditional suture and reconstructive techniques can be implemented in this confined surgical site with the use of robotic technology. These advantages may expand the indications of minimally invasive endoscopic approaches to the skull base. Future development and refinement of endonasal robotic instrumentation is critical before applying these techniques in the clinical setting.

REFERENCES

1. Hanna E, DeMonte F, Ibrahim S, et al. Endoscopic resection of sinonasal cancers with and without craniotomy: oncologic results. Arch Otolaryngol Head Neck Surg 2009;135(12):1219–24.
2. Lund V, Howard DJ, Wei WI. Endoscopic resection of malignant tumors of the nose and sinuses. Am J Rhinol 2007;21(1):89–94.
3. Nicolai P, Battaglia P, Bignami M, et al. Endoscopic surgery for malignant tumors of the sinonasal tract and adjacent skull base: a 10-year experience. Am J Rhinol 2008;22(3):308–16.
4. Suriano M, De Vincentiis M, Colli A, et al. Endoscopic treatment of esthesioneuroblastoma: a minimally invasive approach combined with radiation therapy. Otolaryngol Head Neck Surg 2007;136(1):104–7.
5. Shipchandler TZ, Batra PS, Citardi MJ, et al. Outcomes for endoscopic resection of sinonasal squamous cell carcinoma. Laryngoscope 2005;115(11):1983–7.
6. Anand VK, Schwartz TH, Hiltzik DH, et al. Endoscopic transphenoidal pituitary surgery with real-time intraoperative magnetic resonance imaging. Am J Rhinol 2006;20(4):401–5.
7. Schwartz TH, Stieg PE, Anand VK. Endoscopic transsphenoidal pituitary surgery with intraoperative magnetic resonance imaging. Neurosurgery 2006;58(Suppl 1):ONS44–51 [discussion: ONS44–51].
8. Sethi DS, Leong JL. Endoscopic pituitary surgery. Otolaryngol Clin North Am 2006;39(3):563–83, x.
9. Teo C. Application of endoscopy to the surgical management of craniopharyngiomas. Childs Nerv Syst 2005;21(8–9):696–700.
10. Kassam A, Carrau RL, Snyderman CH, et al. Evolution of reconstructive techniques following endoscopic expanded endonasal approaches. Neurosurg Focus 2005;19(1):E8.
11. Kassam A, Snyderman CH, Mintz A, et al. Expanded endonasal approach: the rostrocaudal axis. Part I. Crista galli to the sella turcica. Neurosurg Focus 2005; 19(1):E3.
12. Kassam AB, Gardner P, Snyderman C, et al. Expanded endonasal approach: fully endoscopic, completely transnasal approach to the middle third of the clivus, petrous bone, middle cranial fossa, and infratemporal fossa. Neurosurg Focus 2005;19(1):E6.
13. Kassam AB, Snyderman C, Gardner P, et al. The expanded endonasal approach: a fully endoscopic transnasal approach and resection of the odontoid process: technical case report. Neurosurgery 2005;57(Suppl 1):E213 [discussion: E213].
14. Solari D, Magro F, Cappabianca P, et al. Anatomical study of the pterygopalatine fossa using an endoscopic endonasal approach: spatial relations and distances between surgical landmarks. J Neurosurg 2007;106(1):157–63.
15. Basu D, Haughey BH, Hartman JM. Determinants of success in endoscopic cerebrospinal fluid leak repair. Otolaryngol Head Neck Surg 2006;135(5):769–73.
16. Locatelli D, Rampa F, Acchiardi I, et al. Endoscopic endonasal approaches for repair of cerebrospinal fluid leaks: nine-year experience. Neurosurgery 2006; 58(4 Suppl 2):ONS-246–56 [discussion: ONS-256–7].
17. Weinstein GS, O'Malley BW Jr, Snyder W, et al. Transoral robotic surgery: supraglottic partial laryngectomy. Ann Otol Rhinol Laryngol 2007;116(1):19–23.
18. Hanna EY, Holsinger C, DeMonte F, et al. Robotic endoscopic surgery of the skull base: a novel surgical approach. Arch Otolaryngol Head Neck Surg 2007; 133(12):1209–14.

19. Kupferman ME, Demonte F, Levine N, et al. Feasibility of a robotic surgical approach to reconstruct the skull base. Skull Base 2011;21(2):79–82.
20. Cappabianca P, Cavallo LM, de Divitiis O, et al. Endoscopic pituitary surgery. Pituitary 2008;11(4):385–90.
21. Liu JK, Weiss MH, Couldwell WT. Surgical approaches to pituitary tumors. Neurosurg Clin N Am 2003;14(1):93–107.
22. Kupferman M, Demonte F, Holsinger FC, et al. Transantral robotic access to the pituitary gland. Otolaryngol Head Neck Surg 2009;141(3):413–5.
23. O'Malley BW Jr, Weinstein GS. Robotic anterior and midline skull base surgery: preclinical investigations. Int J Radiat Oncol Biol Phys 2007;69(Suppl 2):S125–8.
24. Ozer E, Waltonen J. Transoral robotic nasopharyngectomy: a novel approach for nasopharyngeal lesions. Laryngoscope 2008;118(9):1613–6.
25. Wei WI, Ho WK. Transoral robotic resection of recurrent nasopharyngeal carcinoma. Laryngoscope 2010;120(10):2011–4.
26. McCool RR, Warren FM, Wiggins RH 3rd, et al. Robotic surgery of the infratemporal fossa utilizing novel suprahyoid port. Laryngoscope 2010;120(9):1738–43.
27. O'Malley BW Jr, Weinstein GS. Robotic skull base surgery: preclinical investigations to human clinical application. Arch Otolaryngol Head Neck Surg 2007; 133(12):1215–9.
28. Hadad G, Bassagasteguy L, Carrau RL, et al. A novel reconstructive technique after endoscopic expanded endonasal approaches: vascular pedicle nasoseptal flap. Laryngoscope 2006;116(10):1882–6.
29. Leong JL, Citardi MJ, Batra PS. Reconstruction of skull base defects after minimally invasive endoscopic resection of anterior skull base neoplasms. Am J Rhinol 2006;20(5):476–82.
30. Mehta RP, Cueva RA, Brown JD, et al. What's new in skull base medicine and surgery? Skull Base Committee report. Otolaryngol Head Neck Surg 2006;135(4): 620–30.
31. Kassam AB, Carrau RL, Snyderman CH, et al. Endoscopic reconstruction of the cranial base using a pedicled nasoseptal flap. Neurosurgery 2008;63(1 Suppl 1): ONS44–53.

Robotic Facelift Thyroidectomy

Michael C. Singer, MD[a], David J. Terris, MD[b],*

KEYWORDS

- Thyroidectomy • Robotic • Robotic thyroidectomy • Remote access

KEY POINTS

- Robotic facelift thyroidectomy (RFT) uses a facelift incision in the postauricular area to provide entry to the thyroid compartment.
- In order to achieve excellent results with RFT, proper patient selection is critical.
- One difference between RFT and the axillary-based approaches is the ease of positioning required during the surgery.
- RFT has been shown to be a feasible, remote access thyroidectomy approach that offers patients excellent cosmetic outcomes.
- Continued efforts to refine the technique, along with robotic innovations, may expand the indications and benefits of RFT.

INTRODUCTION

The performance of thyroid surgery has changed greatly over the last decade. Incorporating principles and techniques from other surgical fields, a range of minimally invasive and minimal incision thyroidectomy procedures have been developed. The most widely adopted of these is the minimally invasive video-assisted thyroidectomy, described and refined by Miccoli and colleagues.[1] These minimally invasive thyroidectomy techniques are designed to minimize dissection and tissue trauma, leading to decreased postoperative pain and faster recovery times. At the same time, incisions as small as 2 cm can now be used to perform thyroid surgery. When properly placed in the neck, this type of incision typically heals with excellent cosmetic results. Nonetheless, for some patients, any cervical scar is undesirable, including patients with a predisposition to the development of keloids or hypertrophic scars. As a result,

Disclosure: Dr D.J. Terris has directed a series of thyroid courses sponsored by Johnson and Johnson.
[a] Division of Thyroid & Parathyroid Surgery, Department of Otolaryngology, Henry Ford Hospital, 2799 West Grand Boulevard, Detroit, MI 48202, USA; [b] Department of Otolaryngology, GRU Thyroid Center, Georgia Regents University, 1120 Fifteenth Street, BP-4109, Augusta, GA 30912-4060, USA
* Corresponding author.
E-mail address: dterris@gru.edu

surgeons have sought to develop remote access thyroidectomy techniques in which the thyroid compartment is approached from an incision not in the cervical region. These operations result in less conspicuous, noncervical scars.

Many remote access techniques, some endoscopic and others robot assisted, have been described. The most popular of these use the axilla as the access point to the thyroid compartment.[2–5] Robotic facelift thyroidectomy (RFT), uses a facelift incision in the postauricular area to provide entry to the thyroid compartment. This technique was developed based on the notion that this approach would be less invasive, easier to learn, and perhaps safer than the axillary-based approaches.[6,7] RFT consequently is a hybrid approach that integrates important components of traditional thyroid surgery with several innovative principles, including use of the modified facelift incision, the integration of the da Vinci robot (Intuitive Surgical Inc, Sunnyvale, CA), and the use of a fixed retractor system as described by Chung[2]. RFT has now been shown to be feasible and safe and an increasing number of institutions have begun to offer it to select patients.[8] This article describes the indications, technical details, outcomes, and potential complications of RFT.

TREATMENT GOALS

RFT is designed to avoid a cervical incision and achieve thyroidectomy results (both complication rates and completeness of resection) that match those of conventional and minimally invasive thyroidectomy approaches. Although some investigators suggest that the use of the robot in remote access procedures makes them minimally invasive and safer, these claims are difficult to justify. Patients undergoing RFT should understand that this technique offers cosmetic benefits in the context of safely performed thyroid surgery. The goal of RFT (or any remote access procedure) is not to be minimally invasive.

PREOPERATIVE PLANNING AND SPECIAL EQUIPMENT

In order to achieve excellent results with RFT proper patient selection is critical. Appropriate indications and contraindications are shown in **Table 1**.

In RFT, the first phase of the surgery, creating the operative pocket, is completed under direct vision. The surgical robot is then docked and the thyroidectomy begun. To complete the initial phase of the surgery a standard tray of head and neck instruments is needed. In addition, a series of progressively longer retractors and forceps is necessary to facilitate dissection as the pocket is developed inferiorly. An extralong tip electrocautery tip is also helpful during this step of RFT.

Once the operative pocket is created it is maintained by a fixed retractor system that elevates the myocutaneous flap. A second retractor is needed to laterally retract the sternocleidomastoid muscle (SCM). The da Vinci S or Si robot (Intuitive Surgical Inc, Sunnyvale, CA) is used to complete the excision.

Table 1 RFT	
Indications	**Contraindications**
Presumed benign disease	Substernal extension
Nodules ≤4 cm	Likely or known carcinoma
Unilateral surgery	Previous neck surgery
Patient desire to avoid cervical incision	Morbidly obese

dotracheal tube, the patient is
of hair is clipped along the
nd draping, the table is placed
the side of surgery to improve

f the SCM. The surgery pro-
. **2**).[9] The first structure iden-
Dissection is then continued
ernal jugular vein is encoun-
to facilitate access. Recog-
serves as the landmark for
yroid compartment. By dis-
, the sternohyoid and ster-
en reflected from lateral to
omohyoid muscle is most
erally. A malleable retractor
ing retractor (Marina Med-
flap and maintain the oper-
SCM laterally.
Excision of the gland then
during the open phase of
The superior pole is then
the inferior border of the
erior laryngeal nerve can
r parathyroid gland may
tion and identification of
erior constrictor muscle
le from the cricoid carti-
be used as a landmark

the ease of posi-
perating table in
ured in place and
hesia team should
s turned 30° away
n of the neck during
ntralateral to the side

s are placed. At this
cart is positioned on
d parallel to the long
arm is positioned first,
, or angled slightly up-
and a Harmonic device
ominant arm. These de-
er to minimize collisions
ch a way that they create

at the robotic console. A
retracting as necessary.

sition for the incision the pa-
celift incision is placed in the
(**Fig. 1**). The descending limb
this portion of the incision is
om the frontal view, no part of
incision, needed in the unlikely
ell.

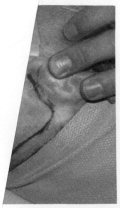

ritical landmarks are
, and the omohyoid
ift thyroidectomy: II.
ission.)

the occipital hairline. This incision is
n Terris DJ, Singer MC, Seybt MW. Robotic
chnical considerations. Surg Laparosc Endosc
)

Following intubation with an electromyographic en
positioned as described earlier. Approximately 1 cn
descending limb of the incision. After sterile prepping a
in reverse Trendelenburg position and turned away from
ergonomics for the operative surgeon.

The incision is made and carried down to the level
ceeds by identifying a series of anatomic structures (Fig
tified is the SCM, followed by the greater auricular nerve
inferiorly along the anterior surface of the SCM. The ex
tered and is typically reflected dorsally or can be ligated
nition of the omohyoid muscle is important because it
the underlying strap muscles and the entry point to the tl
secting and then retracting the omohyoid muscle ventral
nothyroid muscles are exposed. These muscles are th
medial, exposing the upper pole of the thyroid gland. Th
readily seen by retracting the anterior border of the SCM lat
is helpful to accomplish this. A modified version of the Ch
ical, Sunrise, FL) is then used to retract the muscle and skin
ative pocket. A second fixed retractor is used to retract th

At this point the robot is positioned as described earlier.
begins. The superior pedicle of the gland, which is exposed
the surgery, is ligated using the Harmonic device (**Fig. 3**).
reflected ventrally and blunt dissection is used to delineate
inferior constrictor muscle (the external branch of the sup
be seen running along this muscle). In this area the superic
be identified and reflected posteriorly. At this point, explora
the recurrent laryngeal nerve at its entry underneath the in
is achieved (**Fig. 4**). The origin of the inferior constrictor musc
lage can often be visualized. If observed, this oblique line can

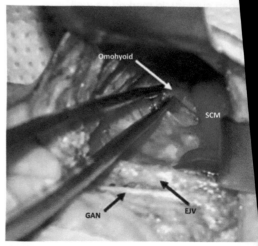

Fig. 2. After a right-sided operative pocket has been developed the c
shown. The great auricular nerve (GAN), external jugular vein (EJV), SCM
muscle are indicated. (*From* Terris DJ, Singer MC, Seybt MW. Robotic facel
Clinical feasibility and safety. Laryngoscope 2011;121(8):1638; with perm

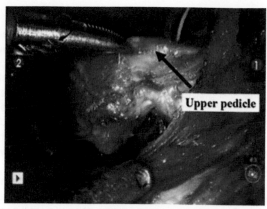

Fig. 3. After the robot is deployed the superior pedicle vessels can be mobilized and ligated. A left-sided superior pedicle is shown just before division. The head of the patient is to the right. (*From* Terris DJ, Singer MC, Seybt MW. Robotic facelift thyroidectomy: II. Clinical feasibility and safety. Laryngoscope 2011;121(8):1638; with permission.)

for identifying the recurrent nerve, because the entry point of the nerve is approximately 1 cm lateral to this line. The nerve is then dissected inferiorly. The tissue medial to this, including the ligament of Berry, may then be safely divided using the Harmonic device. The thyroid isthmus is transected and the middle thyroid vein is ligated. The inferior parathyroid gland is identified and dissected from the thyroid gland, and the inferior pole vessels are ligated. The thyroid gland can then be fully dissected from the trachea and retrieved. The surgeon can elect to stimulate the recurrent nerve a final time at this point. The robotic arms and patient cart are then withdrawn.

After thorough irrigation and inspection of the thyroid bed and surgical pocket, Surgicel (Ethicon Inc, Somerville, NJ) is placed in the thyroid compartment. The wound is then closed in layers. No drain is placed.

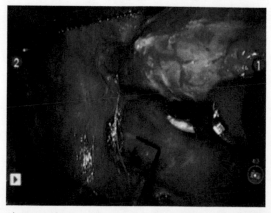

Fig. 4. The recurrent laryngeal nerve is sought after the superior pedicle has been ligated and the superior parathyroid gland mobilized. A probe is shown stimulating a left-sided nerve. The patient's head is to the right and feet to the left. The robotic forceps are retracting the thyroid lobe medially. (*From* Terris DJ, Singer MC, Seybt MW. Robotic facelift thyroidectomy: II. Clinical feasibility and safety. Laryngoscope 2011;121(8):1639; with permission.)

POTENTIAL COMPLICATIONS AND MANAGEMENT

In addition to the potential complications of any form of thyroid surgery, RFT has some risks that exist because of the specific nature of this technique. Although only a limited number of RFTs have been performed, to date the rates of recurrent laryngeal nerve injury and hypoparathyroidism with this surgery have been excellent.[10]

As described earlier, the greater auricular nerve is encountered during the dissection of the operative pocket. Efforts should be made to preserve this nerve. However, even if intact, patients experience a temporary hypesthesia in the distribution of this nerve. Patients should be clearly advised of this potential problem before surgery, but can be reassured that this sensation typically resolves over weeks to months (even when the nerve has been transected).

Because of the large area of dissection in RFT compared with minimally invasive thyroidectomy, the risk of seroma formation exists. Although meticulous hemostasis can likely limit the risk of hematomas and seromas, they may still occur. Most of these do not require intervention and routine aspiration is not advised.

Compared with patients undergoing minimally invasive thyroidectomy, patients seem to have higher levels of pain after RFT. In addition, the recovery time in these patients seems longer. Both of these factors should be acknowledged to patients before surgery.

POSTPROCEDURAL CARE AND RECOVERY

Postoperative care of patients having RFT is the same as for those undergoing conventional minimally invasive or endoscopic thyroidectomy. After observation for several hours in the recovery room, patients are discharged home. As with all patients

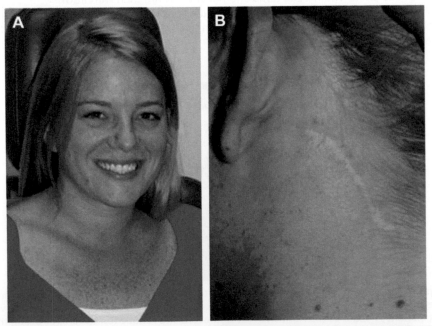

Fig. 5. Frontal view of a patient 1 year after undergoing a bilateral RFT (A). The left-sided postauricular scar (B).

having thyroid surgery, those having RFT are instructed to avoid heavy lifting and exercise for 2 weeks after surgery. Patients follow up as per the surgeon's routine.

OUTCOMES

Clinical outcomes have been excellent. The largest series reported to date includes 45 RFT procedures, including 6 staged bilateral procedures.[10] The average operative time for a lobectomy was 138 minutes in this series. In this report there were 2 seromas (not requiring intervention) and 2 cases of temporary recurrent nerve paresis. There were no cases of permanent laryngeal nerve injury or hypoparathyroidism. Because the postauricular wound is completely hidden (particularly in women with long hair) cosmetic results are superb (**Fig. 5**).

SUMMARY

RFT is still early in its clinical development. It has been shown to be a feasible remote access thyroidectomy approach that offers patients excellent cosmetic outcomes. Continued efforts to refine the technique, along with robotic innovations, may expand the indications and benefits of RFT.

REFERENCES

1. Miccoli P, Berti P, Materazzi G, et al. Results of video-assisted parathyroidectomy: single institution's 6-year experience. World J Surg 2004;28(12):1216–8.
2. Kang SW, Jeong JJ, Nam KH, et al. Robot-assisted endoscopic thyroidectomy for thyroid malignancies using a gasless transaxillary approach. J Am Coll Surg 2009;209(2):e1–7.
3. Kuppersmith RB, Holsinger FC. Robotic thyroid surgery: An initial 474 experience with North American patients. Laryngoscope 2011;475(3):521–6.
4. Luginbuhl A, Schwartz DM, Sestokas AK, et al. Detection of evolving injury to the brachial plexus during transaxillary robotic thyroidectomy. Laryngoscope 2012; 122(1):110–5.
5. Aliyev S, Taskin HE, Agcaoglu O, et al. Robotic transaxillary total thyroidectomy through a single axillary incision. Surgery 2013;153(5):705–10.
6. Terris DJ, Singer MC. Qualitative and quantitative differences between 2 robotic thyroidectomy techniques. Otolaryngol Head Neck Surg 2012;147(1):20–5.
7. Singer MC, Seybt MW, Terris DJ. Robotic facelift thyroidectomy: I. Pre-clinical simulation and morphometric assessment. Laryngoscope 2011;121(8):1631–5.
8. Terris DJ, Singer MC, Seybt MW. Robotic facelift thyroidectomy: II. Clinical feasibility and safety. Laryngoscope 2011;121(8):1636–41.
9. Terris DJ, Singer MC, Seybt MW. Robotic facelift thyroidectomy: patient selection and technical considerations. Surg Laparosc Endosc Percutan Tech 2011;21(4): 237–42.
10. White LC, Singer MC, Terris DJ. Robotic facelift thyroidectomy. Op Tech Oto 2013;24(2):120–5.

Robotic Approaches to the Neck

Yoon Woo Koh, MD, PhD*, Eun Chang Choi, MD, PhD

KEYWORDS

- Robot • Neck dissection • Head and neck cancer • Lymph node metastasis
- Retroauricular incision • Modified facelift incision

KEY POINTS

- Neck dissection (ND) is performed for patients with head and neck squamous cell carcinoma and results in improved regional disease control as well as disease-specific survival.
- When performed through a conventional transcervical approach, ND leaves a visible scar on the neck, regardless of the size of the incision.
- In the past, a scar on the neck has been accepted as unavoidable.
- This article introduces our surgical technique to perform a standard ND while transposing the external scar by using the robotic system via a modified facelift or retroauricular approach.

OVERVIEW

Conventional head and neck surgery for neck dissection (ND) as well as for benign tumors is performed via transcervical incision. However, this conventional approach leaves a prominent scar on the neck, regardless of size. Considering the usual young age of patients with benign neck masses, easily visible scars might have a greater psychological impact on the patients than physicians assume, especially in young women.[1] Therefore, in recent years, innovations in surgical technique have provided several new approaches to hide visible scars by modifying the surgical techniques and using remote access.[2–8] Such efforts have resulted in endoscopic thyroidectomy techniques, and we previously reported our experience of a unilateral axillobreast approach.[9,10] Clinical trials to make scars invisible have extended to other benign cervical lesions, and several investigators have reported the resection of the submandibular gland (SMG) or branchial cleft cyst using the retroauricular (RA) approach with or without an endoscope.[3–8] The retroauricular, or facelift, approach showed good cosmetic effects because the scar was hidden behind the auricle and hair. We recently applied robotics to benign cervical lesions. We reported the feasibility of robot-assisted SMG resection and the Sistrunk operation via an RA approach.[11–13]

Department of Otorhinolaryngology, Yonsei University College of Medicine, 50 Yonseo-ro, Sedaemun-gu, Seoul 120-752, South Korea
* Corresponding author.
E-mail address: ywkohent@yuhs.ac

Otolaryngol Clin N Am 47 (2014) 433–454
http://dx.doi.org/10.1016/j.otc.2014.02.002
0030-6665/14/$ – see front matter © 2014 Elsevier Inc. All rights reserved.

oto.theclinics.com

Since the advent of surgical robotics a few years ago, transoral robotic surgery (TORS) has been actively applied worldwide in head and neck cancer surgery.[14–19] Furthermore, various endoscope-assisted or robot-assisted minimally invasive approaches have been developed and applied to head and neck diseases. Since 2010, our institution has reported the feasibility of robot-assisted ND (RAND) for patients with cN+ necks as well as cN0 necks.[20–31] At first, RAND was performed via the transaxillary and retroauricular (TARA) approach to remove cervical lymphatics from levels I to V.[30] However, through accumulation of surgical experience of RAND, we realized that the operation can be conducted with no difficulty through the RA or modified facelift (MFL) approaches only. Hence, the RA or MFL approach is now considered sufficient when performing RAND in head and neck cancers. This article presents our novel surgical technique of RAND as well as benign neck mass excision via RA or MFL incisions.

TREATMENT GOALS

The authors' hypothesis is that this procedure can produce better cosmetic satisfaction without significant surgical morbidity, but maintain the same quality and standards as in the conventional approach to ND. First and foremost, the procedure should guarantee complete removal of the lesion with acceptable feasibility compared with the conventional external approach. Next, such an approach might also provide patients with better cosmetic results after surgery. The RA approach can be a representative technique to study remote access to the neck, camouflaging the scar in the retroauricular hairline.

Although complications after conventional ND (CND) are uncommon, RAND may improve postoperative cervical wound problems such as fibrotic band formation and wound dehiscence, which are occasionally encountered in a cervical incision. If there is any skin dehiscence, the risk of great vessel exposure leading to fatal bleeding is low, as can be anticipated in conventional transcervical wounds. In addition, postoperative lymphedema can be avoided and the chance of developing wound healing problems after radiotherapy is less because the skin incision site is located far from the radiation field and normal lymphatic drainage are not disturbed. Most advantages of RAND rest on the incision being remotely placed. Considering the area of dissection, it is not more invasive than the traditional transcervical ND. The robotic system merely helps the surgeon to dissect the lymphatic tissue where access is troublesome. A considerable portion of RAND is performed under the gross vision (levels IIa, IIb, III, and Va). From the results of the present study, the numbers of lymph nodes retrieved for each type of RAND were comparable with its conventional counterpart. The combined treatment using TORS and RAND can be of maximal benefit to the patient in terms of cosmesis and postoperative function.

PREOPERATIVE PLANNING AND SPECIAL EQUIPMENT
Patient Selection

The body mass index (BMI [kg/m^2]) and length and circumference of the neck should be considered because they may affect the difficulty and duration of the procedure. There is no absolute contraindication regarding the body habitus or BMI. With more than 100 cases of RAND, we could successfully accomplish the planned procedures without conversion to the CND regardless of BMI. Obesity is not an absolute contraindication to the surgery, but the possible prolongation of operation time should be explained to the patient. Because RAND requires longer operation time than the conventional technique, patients in old age or with comorbidities should be carefully selected.

Every patient should be informed about the procedure, including both the advantages and the disadvantages of RAND and all other options, including CND, and chemoradiotherapy should be suggested. Informed consent should include this, elucidating the possibility of conversion to CND.

Precautions for Anesthesia

For flap elevation and upper ND under direct vision, the operator should be seated near the head of the patient looking cephalocaudally. The endotracheal tube should be directed to the contralateral side and connected to the ventilator, which is located near the patient's feet, 180° from the typical setup. Risks of any other anesthesia-related complications or difficulties for intubation and anesthesia are not specifically increased with this procedure. The airway is not naturally compromised or disturbed in any way through this procedure.

Special Equipment

1. Retractors for skin flap elevation
   - Skin hook.
   - Army-Navy retractor.
   - Right-angle breast retractor.
   - Self-retaining retractor (Sangdosa Inc, Seoul) (**Fig. 1**).
2. Instruments for dissection under direct vision
   - Monopolar cautery tips with variable length (spatula tip is preferred).
   - Harmonic curved shears (Harmonic Ace 23E; Ethicon Endo-Surgery, Cincinnati, OH).
   - DeBakey forceps or Russian forceps.
   - Yankauer suction (see **Fig. 1**).
3. Robotic instrument (da Vinci Robotic System, Intuitive Surgical Inc, Sunnyvale, CA)
   - Twelve-millimeter, 30° face-down endoscope (Intuitive Surgical Inc, Sunnyvale, CA).
   - Five-millimeter, Maryland forceps (Intuitive Surgical Inc, Sunnyvale, CA).
   - Five-millimeter, Harmonic curved shears (Intuitive Surgical Inc, Sunnyvale, CA).
   - Eight-millimeter, ProGrasp forceps (Intuitive Surgical Inc, Sunnyvale, CA): installed at left or right arm depending on the side of ND. It could be substituted by an endoscopic alligator forceps manipulated by a patient-side assistant.
4. Vessel ligation system
   - Hem-o-lok Ligation System (Teleflex Inc, Research Triangle Park, NC).

A   **B**

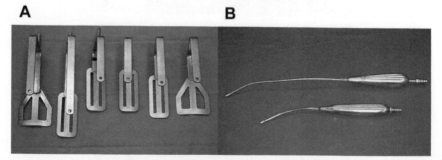

Fig. 1. Self-retaining retractor and Yankauer suction. (*A*) The 2 retractors on the left are Chung retractors used for endoscopic or robotic thyroidectomy and the 4 on the right are self-developed retractors for ND via retroauricular approach or modified facelift incision. (*B*) New self-developed Yankauer suction with long or short length. (*Courtesy of* Sangdosa Inc, Seoul, South Korea; with permission.)

PATIENT AND ROBOT POSITIONING
Positioning of the Patient

The patient is set in a supine position with the neck slightly extended by inserting a soft pillow under the shoulder and with the head rotated toward the contralateral side (**Fig. 2**). The neck is sometimes relaxed in its natural position and not extended.

Positioning of the Robot

After sufficient working space is acquired and upper ND under direct vision is complete, the robotic system is introduced. After placing the foot end of the surgical bed 180° from the anesthesia team, the patient is placed in a supine position, and the manipulator cart and surgical bed are located 30° from the head on each side. A face-down 30° endoscope is used for visualization of the surgical field and 2 robotic instrument arms, equipped at either side of the endoscopic arm with 5-mm Maryland forceps and 5-mm Harmonic curved shears respectively, are used throughout the operation (**Fig. 3**). A patient-side assistant can facilitate the robotic dissection by exposing the surgical field using an Army-Navy retractor or Yankauer suction.

PROCEDURE
Robot-assisted Neurogenic Tumor Excision

The patient is placed in the supine position, the neck is extended, and the head is rotated to the contralateral side. A skin incision is made behind the auricle starting from the lower end of the retroauricular sulcus, moved upward to the midpoint of the sulcus, and then smoothly angulated downward 0.5 cm inside the hairline. Care should

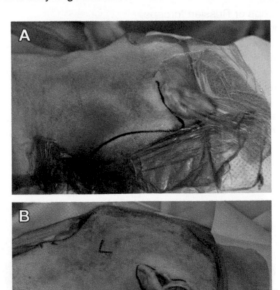

Fig. 2. Position of the patient and design of the skin incision. (*A*) A retroauricular incision. (*B*) A modified facelift incision.

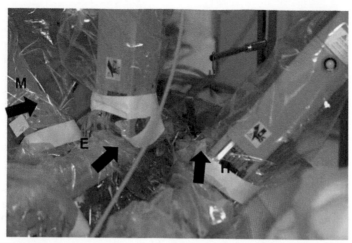

Fig. 3. Position of the robot and placement of the robotic arms for the left-side ND. An endoscopic arm and 2 instrument arms are inserted through an RA incision. E, a face-down 30° endoscope; H, 5 mm Harmonic curved shears; M, 5-mm Maryland forceps. (*Courtesy of Ethicon, Cincinnati, OH; with permission.*)

be taken to avoid damaging the hair follicles during the skin incision and subcutaneous dissection. The subplatysmal skin flap is elevated just above the sternocleidomastoid muscle and carried in an anterior and inferior direction using a monopolar coagulator under direct vision. Special attention is paid to preserve the great auricular nerve and other sensory nerves. When the mass is fully exposed, a self-retaining retractor is introduced, and the skin flap is raised using a lifting device to create a working space (**Fig. 4**).

The da Vinci S Robotic System (Intuitive Surgical Inc, Sunnyvale, CA) is deployed, with a 30°-down dual endoscope in the center, a Maryland forceps in the nondominant hand, and a Metzenbaum scissors (PK Dissecting Forceps) in the dominant hand of the robotic arm. If needed, ProGrasp forceps (Intuitive Surgical) may be installed to enhance the dissection of tumor. Careful enucleation of schwannoma should be done by dissection of the carotid space between the carotid artery and the internal jugular vein (IJV) with dissecting forceps without neural damage under magnification. Attention should be paid to prevent the injury to the jugular vein, the carotid artery, and other nervous systems. **Figs. 5** and **6** show this technique used for a neurogenic tumor, which should be identified and dissected to preserve the neural function.

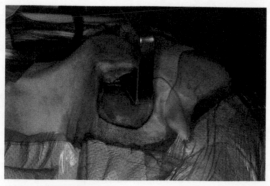

Fig. 4. Setup of a self-retaining retractor.

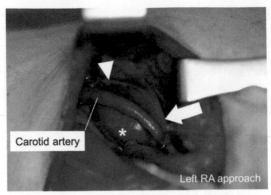

Fig. 5. Exposure of a neurogenic tumor of poststyloid parapharyngeal space. Asterisk, neurogenic tumor; white arrow, hypoglossal nerve; white arrowhead, ansa hypoglossi.

Robot-assisted SMG Excision

The procedure for robotic dissection of SMG is similar to that for endoscopic SMG excision but the instrumentation of the robotic system makes the dissection more convenient. The 30° dual-channel endoscope provides a three-dimensional magnified view and the highly articulated wrist and 360° motion of the robotic arm controlled by the surgeons facilitates the dissection. Dissection begins at the lower border of the SMG. Dissection is conducted using a Harmonic curved shears or a monopolar cautery according to the surgeons preference. The Maryland dissector controlled by the surgeon and a Yankauer suction handled by a bedside assistant provides traction and countertraction, which facilitates the dissection between the SMG and surrounding

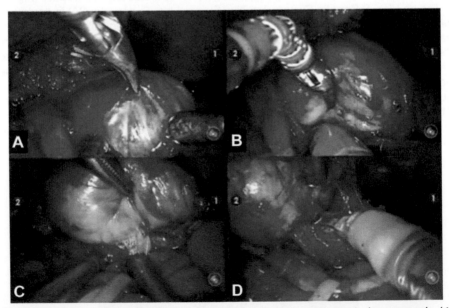

Fig. 6. Robot-assisted excision of the neurogenic tumor via a retroauricular approach. (A) Identification of the tumor capsule. (B, C) Subcapsular dissection of the tumor. (D) Note that enucleation of the tumor was accomplished with preserving the nerve sheath of the vagus. (*Courtesy of* Intuitive Surgical Inc, Sunnyvale, CA; with permission.)

tissues. Compared with the 2 arms of endoscopic dissection for traction and dissection, robotic dissection provides 4 hands at most (2 robotic arms and the 2 arms of the bedside assistant). The bedside assistant can use the Yankauer suction, endoscopic dissector, or an Army-Navy retractor to aid the surgical exposure and dissection. Traction and countertraction in robotic dissection not only facilitate the dissection of the SMG but also may prevent injury to the gland or the tumor, which may occur during dissection with excessive traction only. The proximal facial artery is ligated with the Harmonic curved shears or vascular clips, as is done with endoscopic dissection (**Fig. 7**A). The lingual nerve is separated from the submandibular ganglion with monopolar cautery or the Harmonic curved shears (see **Fig. 7**B), and the Wharton duct is ligated with a vascular clip or a Harmonic curved shears (see **Fig. 7**C). The lingual nerve and hypoglossal nerve are well preserved, and dissection should be performed closely attached to the surface of the gland to prevent thermal injury to these structures (see **Fig. 7**D). The capsule of the intraglandular mass is carefully preserved to prevent tumor spillage.

Robot-assisted Excision of a Thyroglossal Duct Cyst (Sistrunk Operation)

After flap elevation through the retroauricular incision in the plane of the subplatysmal layer, the cystic lesion is identified beneath the superficial layer of the strap muscles. The fibrofatty tissue at the anterior neck is divided using a 5-mm Maryland forceps and 5-mm spatula monopolar cautery for midline identification. The cystic lesion is carefully dissected away from the surrounding fibroconnective tissue and muscle. After identifying the left great horn of the hyoid bone, the tumor is carefully dissected

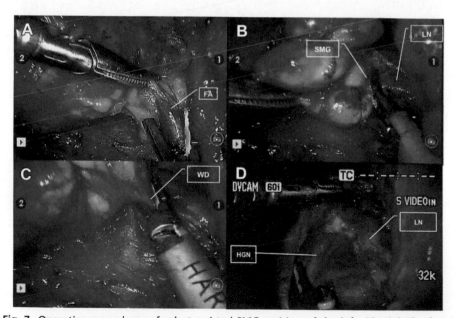

Fig. 7. Operative procedures of robot-assisted SMG excision of the left side. (*A*) The facial artery (FA) is ligated using the Harmonic scalpel during robotic SMG excision of the left side. (*B*) The submandibular ganglion (SMG) is ligated using the Harmonic scalpel during robotic SMG excision of the left side (LN, lingual nerve). (*C*) The Wharton duct (WD) is ligated using the Harmonic scalpel during robotic SMG excision of the left side. (*D*) The SMG of the left side is removed and the hypoglossal nerve (HN) and the LN are preserved. (*Courtesy of* Ethicon, Cincinnati, OH; with permission.)

from the surrounding tissue and mobilized (**Fig. 8**A). Following the skeletonization of the ipsilateral hyoid bone, a bone cutter is introduced through the retroauricular port and the ipsilateral hyoid bone is resected by an assistant (see **Fig. 8**B). After that, infrahyoid muscles together with fibroconnective tissue is dissected and freed from the mass (see **Fig. 8**C). Further extension of the thyroglossal duct should be checked beyond the hyoid bone. Further dissection is then done to the contralateral side using monopolar cautery and the contralateral side of the hyoid bone is cut as well (see **Fig. 8**D). In addition, careful dissection should be done to remove the main mass together with the resected hyoid bone.

Robot-assisted Selective ND (Level I–III)

Skin incision design
An MFL or RA incision is designed according to the surgical extent and types of surgery. The RA incision is made behind the auricle starting from the lower end of the retroauricular sulcus and moving upward to the midpoint of the sulcus, and then smoothly angulated downward 0.5 cm inside the hairline (see **Fig. 2**A). An MFL incision is extended from the RA incision to the natural preauricular fold and continued behind the tragus (see **Fig. 2**B). At first, the MFL approach was mostly chosen because it provided a wider and higher working space for the robotic instrument arms than the RA

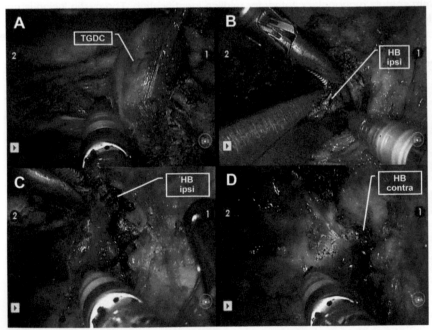

Fig. 8. Operative procedures of robot-assisted Sistrunk operation. (*A*) The fibrofatty tissue at the anterior neck is divided using a 5-mm Maryland forceps and a 5-mm spatula monopolar cautery for midline identification. (*B*) After identifying the left great horn of the hyoid bone, the tumor is carefully dissected from the surrounding tissue and mobilized (HB ipsi, ipsilateral hyoid bone). (*C*) After resecting the ipsilateral hyoid bone, infrahyoid muscles together with fibroconnective tissue is dissected and freed away from the mass. (*D*) Further dissection is done to the contralateral side using the monopolar cautery and the contralateral side of the hyoid bone is cut as well. HB contra, contralateral hyoid bone; TGDC, thyroglossal duct cyst.

approach. However, as our experience with RAND increased, we realized that the RA approach could create a sufficient working space for robotic arms without preauricular incision. The RA approach is now mainly used for RAND.

Skin flap elevation

A subplatysmal skin flap is elevated just above the sternocleidomastoid (SCM) muscle using monopolar cautery under direct vision and is continued to the midline of the anterior neck, superiorly to the inferior margin of the mandible, and inferiorly to the level of omohyoid muscle. Two assistants pull the skin flap with the Army-Navy retractor or right-angle breast retractor. The greater auricular nerve and external jugular vein should be preserved superficial to the SCM muscle (**Fig. 9**). Skin flap elevation below the mandible should be conducted with care not to give thermal injury to the marginal branch of the facial nerve. After identifying the contour of the SMG, the lateral border of the strap muscles should be identified medially and the superior belly of the omohyoid muscle should be identified inferiorly. When sufficient working space is acquired, a self-retaining retractor is applied.

Upper ND under direct vision before docking the robotic arms

Before docking the robotic arms, dissection of fibrofatty tissues accessible under direct vision is performed with CND technique. The marginal branch of the facial nerve is first identified using the distal facial artery and vein as indicators and is preserved by carefully dissecting it from the surrounding fibroadipose tissues and thereby thoroughly dissecting the perifacial lymph nodes. The distal facial artery (**Fig. 10**) and vein are identified along the inferior border of the mandible and ligated with Harmonic curved shears (Harmonic Ace 23E; Ethicon Endo-Surgery, Cincinnati, OH). The lymphofatty tissues inferior to the parotid tail are dissected using a Monopolar coagulator. Dissection of the inferior border of the SMG leads to identification of the posterior belly of the digastric muscle. Fibroadipose tissues are dissected from the anterior surface of the SCM muscle using a monopolar coagulator. Dissection between the inferior border of the digastric muscle and the anterior border of the SCM leads to exposure of the IJV. The transverse process of atlas can be palpated at this area where the spinal accessory nerve usually crosses the IJV. After identifying the spinal accessory nerve and dissecting it, level IIb can be dissected. While preserving the cervical plexus, the fibroadipose tissues of level IIa and III can be dissected toward the carotid sheath using monopolar cautery (**Fig. 11**).

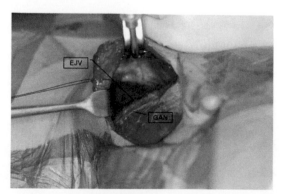

Fig. 9. Skin flap elevation and acquirement of working space for the left-side ND. The greater auricular nerve (GAN) and external jugular vein (EJV) should be preserved superficial to the SCM muscle.

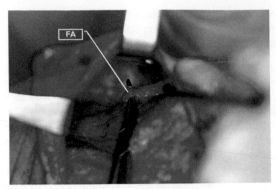

Fig. 10. Distal Facial Artery (FA) and marginal mandibular branch of the facial nerve. The marginal branch of the facial nerve should be identified. The distal FA, located deep to the nerve, may be a good landmark.

RAND technique

Three robotic arms are used, and all three arms are inserted via the retroauricular approach: a 30° dual-channel endoscope (Intuitive Surgical) is placed on the central camera arm, Harmonic curved shears (Intuitive Surgical) or a 5-mm spatula monopolar coagulator is placed on the right arm, and a 5-mm Maryland dissector (Intuitive Surgical) is placed on the left arm of the scope (see **Fig. 3**). In general, ProGrasp forceps can be substituted by endoscopic alligator forceps manipulated by a patient-side assistant.

The robotic dissection begins from level I. Dissection of level I is conducted in a lateral to medial direction. The posterior belly of the digastric muscle is first identified, and then the proximal facial artery is sealed with Harmonic curved shears or double ligated by the assistant with the Hem-o-lok Ligation System (Teleflex Inc, Research Triangle Park, NC) (**Fig. 12A**). While pulling the fibroadipose tissues with the Maryland dissector, level I is dissected from the surrounding muscles (see **Fig. 12B**). The marginal mandibular branch of the facial nerve, lingual nerve, and hypoglossal nerve should be safely preserved during the dissection of the SMG (**Fig. 13A**). After identification of the mylohyoid muscle, the SMG ganglion and the Wharton duct are sealed, with preservation of the hypoglossal and lingual nerve (see **Fig. 12C, D**). The

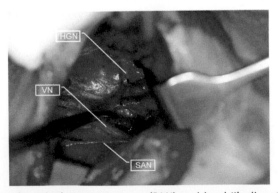

Fig. 11. Identifying the spinal accessory nerve (SAN) and level IIb dissection. The lymphofatty tissues are dissected from the medial border of the sternocleidomastoid muscle and the SAN is traced in the inferior direction. HGN, hypoglossal nerve; VN, vagus nerve.

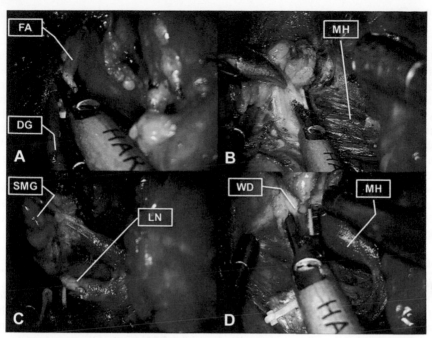

Fig. 12. Level I dissection of the left side. (*A*) Ligation of proximal FA. (*B*) Lymph node dissection from mylohyoid muscle. (*C*) Dissection of submandibular ganglion from lingual nerve. (*D*) WD. The duct is ligated deep to the mylohyoid muscle (MH). DG, posterior belly of digastric muscle; FA, proximal facial artery; MH, mylohyoid muscle. (*Courtesy of* Ethicon, Cincinnati, OH; with permission.)

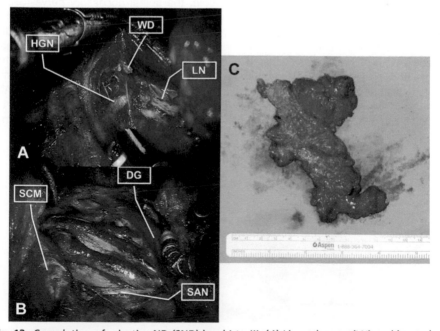

Fig. 13. Completion of selective ND (SND) level I to III. (*A*) Lingual nerve (LN) and hypoglossal nerve (HGN) should be safely preserved during the dissection of SMG. (*B*) Surgical field after SND level I to III. (*C*) Surgical specimen. DG, posterior belly of digastric muscle; SAN, spinal accessary nerve; SCM, sterno-cleidomastoid muscle; WD, Wharton's duct.

submental artery is sealed with Harmonic curved shears. The fibrofatty tissues between both anterior bellies of the digastric muscle (level IA) are detached using Harmonic curved shears. After completing the level I dissection, the fibroadipose tissues of level II and III dissected under direct vision are pulled medially using the Maryland dissector and dissected from the carotid sheath and the IJV. During the level IIa dissection, the hypoglossal nerve can be easily identified and preserved. Dissection is conducted inferiorly to the superior belly of the omohyoid muscle and medially to the lateral border of the strap muscles (see **Fig. 13B**). The superior thyroid artery and ansa cervicalis can be easily identified through the magnified view and preserved. After completing the dissection, the specimen is removed (see **Fig. 13C**). The specimen should be mapped according to each level and sent for biopsy. The surgical field is irrigated, a closed suction drain is inserted posterior to the hairline, and cosmetic skin repair is performed.

Robot-assisted Modified Radical ND (Level I–V or II–V)

Skin incision and flap elevation
When level I is omitted, there is no need to elevate the skin flap as high as the inferior border of the mandible, and the working space must extend to below to the clavicle in order to address levels IV and V. Therefore the skin flap must be elevated more laterally based on the posterior border of the SCM so that the lymph nodes of level V are included. It is helpful if the operator is positioned above the patient's head.

Upper ND under direct vision before docking the robotic arms
Whenever robot-assisted Modified Radical ND (MRND) is to be performed, an effort should be made to preserve the SCM muscle, the spinal accessory nerve (SAN), and the IJV. Dissection is performed along the inferior border of the SMG and the tail of parotid gland, and the posterior belly of the digastric muscle and the IJV should be identified at this point. The SAN can then be identified near the IJV, with the transverse process of the atlas as a landmark. The fascia of the SCM is then opened at the medial border of the SCM and continued as far below as possible to level IV. The lymphofatty tissues are dissected from the medial border of the SCM muscle and the SAN is traced in the inferior direction (**Fig. 14**). The SAN is identified at the lateral border of the SCM muscle (**Fig. 15**). The SAN is traced and skeletonized and the SAN running

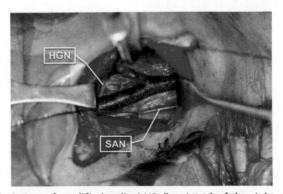

Fig. 14. The surgical view of modified radical ND (level II–V) of the right side. Surgical field after superior traction of the sternocleidomastoid muscle. The SAN is identified near the transverse process of the second cervical spine and traced to the insertion to the trapezius muscle.

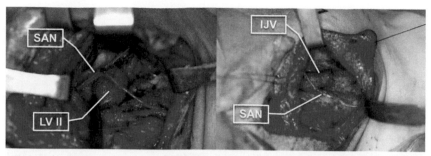

Fig. 15. Levels IIB, VA, IIA, and upper III dissections of the right side. With the upward retraction of the skeletonized SCM muscle, levels IIB, VA, and the lateral aspect to the carotid sheath of IIA and upper III are dissected under direct vision. LV II, level II lymph node.

toward the trapezius at the Erb point of the SCM's posterior border is identified (see **Fig. 15**). The entire SAN from the skull base to the trapezius muscle is identified and skeletonized. Next, the surgeon opens the fascia along the whole lateral border of the SCM, and the fibrofatty tissue is dissected from the inner side of the SCM by elevating it upward using an Army-Navy retractor (see **Fig. 15**). All fibroadipose tissues are dissected off the SCM during this procedure, and care must be taken not to damage the SAN running to the trapezius at this point (see **Fig. 15**). The skeletonized SCM muscle is lifted, and levels IIB, VA, the lateral aspect to the carotid sheath of IIA, and upper III are dissected under direct vision (see **Fig. 15**). With the accumulation of surgical experience, most upper ND including levels IIa and III medial to the carotid sheath can be accomplished under direct vision. A self-retaining retractor (Sangdosa, Seoul, Korea) is then inserted through the working space and the SCM muscle is elevated and is then ready for the robotic arms to be introduced. The sequence of the operation in general, before docking of the robotic arms, is that levels IIb and Va must be dissected first at the lateral portion of the SAN and, after elevating the SCM muscle, some portion of levels IIA and III located lateral to the carotid sheath should be dissected under direct vision (see **Fig. 15**).

RAND technique
Because dissection of levels IV and V is required, the robotic arms must be inserted so that they are addressed toward level IV and V. With superior and medial retraction of level IIb specimen, which has already been dissected, the level IIa dissection is started, in a superior to inferior direction. The hypoglossal nerve is identified and preserved near the carotid bifurcation area. During the level IIa dissection, the superior thyroid and lingual artery are identified and preserved. Next, level III is dissected using the robotic system, again in a superior to inferior direction. Lymphofatty tissue is carefully dissected from the IJV using Harmonic curved shears equipped with robotic arms. Because the skin flap and SCM are already elevated, it is not difficult to dissect level V (posterior to anterior) in cases in which level V dissection is required. In a lateromedial direction, the fibrofatty tissues in level VB are dissected (**Fig. 16**A, B). The omohyoid muscle is identified and cut using Harmonic curved shears. The transverse cervical artery and vein are verified on the floor of level V and the phrenic nerve is identified beneath the transverse cervical vessels (see **Fig. 16**C). The specimen is then retracted superiorly and medially, and level IV dissection is performed. The fibrofatty tissues near the carotid space in level IV are dissected using Harmonic curved shears. The vagus nerve, carotid artery, and jugular vein are identified and preserved by carefully opening the carotid sheath (see **Fig. 16**B). During the dissection of level IV, the

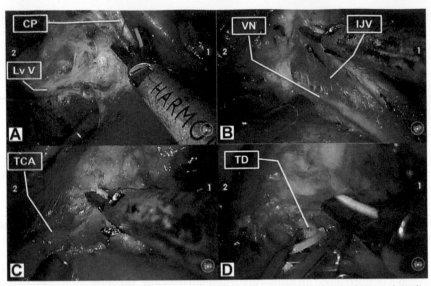

Fig. 16. The surgical view of modified radical ND (level II–V) of the left side. (*A*) Level VB dissection. The fibrofatty tissues in level VB are dissected in a lateromedial direction. (*B*) Carotid sheath dissection. The fibrofatty tissues near the carotid space in level IV is dissected using Harmonic curved shears. (*C*) Identification and preservation of the transverse cervical artery. The transverse cervical artery is verified and the phrenic nerve is located beneath the transverse cervical vessels. (*D*) Ligation of the thoracic duct. The thoracic duct is sealed with Hem-O-Lok to prevent a chyle leakage. CP, cervical plexus; Lv V, level V area; TCA, transverse cervical artery; TD, thoracic duct. (*Courtesy of* Teleflex Medical, Lumberton, NJ; with permission.)

lymphatic or thoracic duct should be ligated using hemoclips or the Hem-o-lok Ligation System to prevent a chyle leakage (see **Fig. 16**D). The branches of the IJV are ligated with Harmonic curved shears or the Hem-o-lok Ligation System. After the ND is complete (**Fig. 17**A), the neck specimens are removed through the MFL or RA

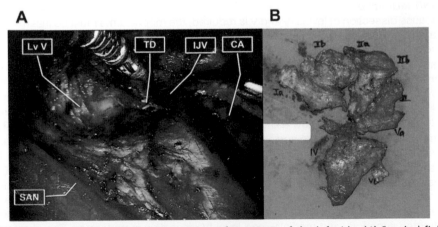

Fig. 17. Surgical field and surgical specimen after MRND of the left side. (*A*) Surgical field after MRND. (*B*) The specimen is removed through the RA or MFL incision. The specimen can be separately removed with a level-by-level strategy. CA, carotid artery; IJV, internal jugular vein; Lv V, level V area; SAN, spinal accessory nerve; TD, thoracic duct.

incision (see **Fig. 17**B). The surgical bed is irrigated with warm saline and bleeding control under both endoscopic view and direct vision should be performed (see **Fig. 17**A). A closed suction drain is placed in the wound and the incision is closed with 4-0 Vicryl and 5-0 nylon sutures.

Potential complications and their management
Potential complications from RAND
- Nerve injury
  - Lingual nerve injury
  - Marginal mandibular branch of facial nerve injury (mouth corner deviation)
  - Vagus nerve injury (vocal cord palsy)
  - Spinal accessary nerve (SAN) injury (spinal accessory nerve syndrome)
  - Hypoglossal nerve injury
  - Phrenic nerve injury
  - Sympathetic nerve injury (Horner syndrome)
- Bleeding/hematoma
- Seroma
- Chyle leakage (lymphatic/thoracic duct injury)
- Wound infection, dehiscence
- Ischemia or necrosis of skin flap

Management of complications
Postoperative bleeding or hematoma Minor bleeding from the skin flap or muscles that may lead to postoperative hematoma may be resolved with conservative management. However, major bleeding, possibly from ligated or clipped vessels, may present as abrupt swelling of the neck. Surgical exploration under general anesthesia should be conducted in such cases. However, significant postoperative bleeding after robot-assisted neck surgery is extremely rare in our experience.

Nerve injury We have experienced several cases of temporary paralysis of the marginal branch of the facial nerve that recovered within 2 to 3 months. Traction or thermal injury to the nerve may cause such a deficit. Therefore, both the surgeon and the assistant should take care to prevent such injury at the inferior border of the mandible. Injury to the hypoglossal nerve, lingual nerve, SAN, vagus nerve, and sympathetic nerve is extremely rare with thorough anatomic understanding of the structures and magnified visualization. To prevent these nerve injuries, comprehensive understanding of the anatomy of the neurovascular structures is essential. Temporary or permanent numbness of ear lobe caused by injury to the greater auricular nerve may be caused by thermal injury to the nerve. However, these nerves may be more vulnerable to dissection with the Harmonic scalpel during RAND rather than during CND. Surgeons should therefore be familiar with the use of the Harmonic scalpel even in conventional neck surgery.

Chyle leakage (lymphatic/thoracic duct injury) The lymphatic duct or thoracic duct is also a thin-walled structure even though the pressure is not high, so great care must be taken when ligating it. After retrieval of an ND specimen, the level IV area should be inspected for any evidence of chyle leakage. If chylous leakage is suspected, hemoclip or Hem-o-lok (Teleflex MED) Ligation System should be applied. We routinely check for chylous leakage with the positive pressure ventilation before finishing the operation.

Ischemia or necrosis of skin flap Such complications may occur at the tip of retro-auricular skin flap because of insufficient blood supply. We have experienced discoloration (ischemic change) but not serious skin necrosis. However, care must be taken that the skin flap does not become too thin. The platysma muscle should be always identified as the skin flap elevation proceeds. Otherwise it may lead to thinning of the skin flap, which could result in postoperative skin necrosis, discoloration, depression, or even penetration of the skin.

Hypertrophic scar or keloid formation Meticulous handling of the skin flap and minimizing of tissue injury during the surgery may be helpful to prevent such complications. Skin closure should be conducted with minimal skin tension after proper suturing of the subcutaneous tissue.

Hair loss along the skin incision Hair loss along the skin incision within the hairline can occur. In order to prevent such situations, beveling the skin incision or placing the incision in front of the hairline might be useful.

Postprocedural care and recovery
Postoperative care may be no different to care after conventional neck surgery. The neck should be closely monitored for any signs of hemorrhage, hematoma, or infection. The closed suction drain can be removed if the drainage amount decreases to less than 20 mL a day. The patient of RAND can be discharged in about a week, 1 day after the suction drain has been removed. Second, any change of skin color or signs of skin flap necrosis should be detected. Third, the possibility of orocervical fistula should be borne in mind when RAND is followed by TORS.

Outcomes and clinical results in the literature
We recently reported our surgical techniques of endoscopic and robot-assisted SMG resection through a retroauricular incision, which were not only feasible but also had excellent cosmetic outcomes, leaving a scar that is hidden by the auricle and hair.[12] The surgical techniques and feasibility of endoscopic sialadenectomy[3,4,6-8] of the SMG have been presented by several other investigators. In our previous feasibility study of robot-assisted SMG resection,[11,12] we proposed that the robot-assisted technique may overcome the limitations of endoscopic instruments, which are rigid and straight and lack the ability to articulate or provide a three-dimensional surgical view. In addition, the ergonomically designed robotic system was more convenient for the surgeon, considering the frequent collision of endoscopic instruments and the inverted hand-eye coordination involved with endoscopic surgery. We recently reported that the surgical outcomes of the two techniques were comparable (**Table 1**).[12] The robot-assisted procedure improved technical convenience for the surgeon but has not shown any significant clinical benefit regarding outcome. We expect that, as experience with the robot-assisted SMG resection accumulates and further innovations of robotic technology are introduced, improved outcomes may be anticipated, including the reduction of operating room time.

RAND is a feasible and safe technique as an elective or therapeutic neck treatment in patients with cN0 and cN+ head and neck squamous cell carcinoma (HNSCC).[20-31] We previously reported the feasibility of robot-assisted supraomohyoid ND for clinically node-negative oral tongue cancer and documented the satisfactory operative parameters obtained (**Table 2**).[27] These findings were the foundation for the rationale for the MRND via the RA or MFL approaches. This RAND technique via a retroauricular or MFL approach may be especially helpful in patients who have undergone TORS or transoral resection to remove a primary lesion because it does not leave a visible scar around the neck. In addition, we think that there are benefits of RAND compared with CND in functional aspects such as subcutaneous induration/fibrosis, lymphedema,

Table 1
Comparison of surgical outcomes between endoscopic and robot-assisted SMG resection through a retroauricular incision

Characteristics	EAR Group (n = 22)	RAR Group (n = 13)	P Value
Length of incision (cm)	8.0 ± 0.3 (7.3–8.5)	8.1 ± 0.3 (7.6–8.8)	.544
Total operation time (min)	66.5 ± 9.1 (50–85)	63.4 ± 6.3 (53–74)	.149
Intraoperative bleeding (mL)	11.0 ± 3.3 (6–19)	9.7 ± 3.1 (5–15)	.252
Amount of drainage (mL)	119.5 ± 34.0 (73–184)	121.5 ± 73.0 (64–351)	.928
Duration of drainage (d)	2.7 ± 0.9 (2–5)	2.9 ± 1.1 (2–6)	.686
Hospital stay (d)	3.8 ± 1.1 (2–6)	3.5 ± 0.9 (2–6)	.453
Complications			.677
Mouth corner deviation[a]	2	1	—
Numbness of auricle	2	1	—
Postoperative seroma	0	1	—
Hypertrophic scar	1	0	—
Cosmetic satisfaction score	4.4 ± 0.5	4.2 ± 0.6	.276

Data are mean ± standard deviation (range) unless otherwise stated.
Abbreviations: EAR, endoscope-assisted resection; RAR, robot-assisted resection.
[a] Temporary in all patients.
Data from Lee HS, Kim D, Lee SY, et al. Robot-assisted versus endoscopic submandibular gland resection via retroauricular approach: a prospective nonrandomized study. Br J Oral Maxillofac Surg 2014;52(2):179–84.

Table 2
Postoperative outcome of robot-assisted and conventional supraomohyoid ND

Variables	Robot-assisted ND (n = 10)	CND (n = 16)	P Value
Operation time (min)	157 ± 18	78 ± 6	.000
Amount of drainage (mL)	258 ± 40	240 ± 38	.286
Duration of drainage (d)	5.6 ± 0.8	5.3 ± 1.6	.241
Hospital stay (d)	9.1 ± 1.6	10.8 ± 5.1	.897
Retrieved LNs	22 ± 4	20 ± 4	.310
Satisfaction of scar	4.0 ± 0.7	2.2 ± 0.8	.000
Complication			
Numbness of earlobe	6	4	.109
Temporary mouth corner deviation	2	2	.625
Shoulder syndrome			
Shoulder droop	0	0	—
Shoulder pain score	2.25	2.29	.872
Shoulder motion score	2.75	2.84	.412
Adjuvant therapy	CCRT (1)	CCRT (2)	—
	RT (2)	RT (2)	—
Median follow-up (month)	6	6	—

Abbreviations: CCRT, concurrent chemoradiation therapy; LN, lymph node; ND, neck dissection; RT, radiation therapy.
Data from Lee HS, Kim WS, Hong HJ, et al. Robot-assisted supraomohyoid neck dissection via a modified face-lift or retroauricular approach in early-stage cN0 squamous cell carcinoma of the oral cavity: a comparative study with conventional technique. Ann Surg Oncol 2012;19(12):3871–8.

incision site sensory disturbance, and objective range of neck motion. Based on the normal anatomic subcutaneous lymphatic channel of the head and neck, the transverse incision in the anterior neck can significantly disrupt lymphatic drainage, which is generally prevented by the use of RA or MFL incisions. We evaluated the functional outcomes of RAND through patient-perceived and objective parameters (Byeon HK & Koh YW, 2014). Regarding motor function, there was no significant difference between the CND and RAND groups, although the patients in both groups showed a tendency to improve in both subjective and objective measurements with time. In terms of the

Table 3 Operative parameters of robot-assisted and CND group			
Characteristics	RAND (n = 20)	CND (n = 33)	P Value
Operation time for ND (min)	186 ± 37	150 ± 23	.000
Estimated blood loss during ND (mL)	259 ± 76	239 ± 71	.354
Amount of drainage (mL)	894 ± 424	794 ± 306	.327
Duration of drainage (d)	9.7 ± 4.0	8.2 ± 2.0	.145
Hospital stay (d)	17.0 ± 8.1	15.5 ± 7.8	.522
Free flap reconstruction	3	8	.503
SCM muscle sacrifice	6	10	1.000
IJV ligation	3	7	.725
Intentional SAN sacrifice	2	3	1.000
Conversion to CND	0	—	—
Perioperative complications			
Seroma	4	5	.715
Hematoma	2	1	.549
Chyle leakage	2	4	1.000
Skin flap necrosis/dehiscence	0	1	1.000
Orocervical fistula[a]	0	2	.521
Lingual nerve injury	0	0	—
Hypoglossal nerve injury	0	0	—
Phrenic nerve palsy	0	0	—
SAN injury[b]	0	1	1.000
Vagus nerve injury	0	0	—
Sympathetic trunk injury	1	0	—
Temporary mouth corner deviation	4	3	.405
Satisfaction of scar	3.6 ± 1.1	2.8 ± 1.1	.023
Adjuvant therapy			
CCRTx	13	21	—
RTx	6	9	—
Median follow-up (mo)	8.0	9.3	.456
Nodal recurrence	0	2	.521

Abbreviations: CCRTx, concurrent chemoradiotherapy; RAND, robot-assisted neck dissection; RTx, radiotherapy; SCM, sternocleidomastoid muscle.
    [a] Orocervical fistula in cases of oropharynx cancer.
    [b] Unexpected SAN injury or resection.
    Data from Kim WS, Byeon HK, Park YM, et al. Therapeutic robot-assisted neck dissection via a retroauricular or modified face lift approach in head and neck cancer: a comparative study with conventional transcervical neck dissection. Head Neck 2013 Dec 24 [Epub ahead of print].

sensory function, postoperative pain score was significantly lower in the RAND group at 12-month follow-up. Hypoesthesia complaints significantly improved with time in the RAND group. Patients in both groups complained of dysesthesia, allodynia, and neuralgia until 12 months after ND. As for the cosmetic outcomes, patient-perceived satisfaction with the wounds was significantly higher in the RAND group. The incidence of lymphedema, subcutaneous induration, and fibrosis was significantly lower and the degree much less in the RAND group.

As our experience with RAND increased, we saw the potential for therapeutic RAND in node-positive patients. We recently reported the comparative results of therapeutic RAND via an RA or MFL approach with CND in HNSCC (**Table 3**).[31] The RAND and CND groups consisted of 20 and 33 patients, respectively. The mean operative time for the RAND group was significantly longer than that of the CND group. The mean number of retrieved lymph nodes in the RAND group was not significantly different from that in the CND group. Based on these results, we speculated that therapeutic RAND via an RA or MFL approach was feasible with satisfactory esthetic results in selected patients with N+ HNSCC. Although this surgical novelty may not be widely applied given the increased costs and long learning curve, the RAND technique via an RA or MFL approach may be successfully applied to selected cases by an experienced surgeon.

SUMMARY

For selected cases, ND via RA or MFL approach seems to provide increased patient satisfaction because of improved cosmesis, and it maintains adequacy of dissection and comparable rates of lymph node harvest. We found increased technical convenience with the robot, which may not be evident from simple comparison of numerical values. The highly articulated robotic arms with 7 degrees of freedom under a three-dimensional magnified view allow the surgeon to manipulate the devices efficiently within the narrow working space.

RAND may be especially helpful in patients who have undergone TORS or transoral resection to remove a primary lesion because it does not leave a visible scar around the neck (**Fig. 18**).[20–31] Moreover, we think that there are benefits of RAND compared with CND in functional aspects such as subcutaneous induration/fibrosis, lymphedema, incision site sensory disturbance, and objective range of neck motion. However, RAND should not be applied for every case for which ND is indicated, because the oncologic safety could be violated in cases of neck nodal metastases with evident extracapsular spread (ECS), including carotid artery encasement. Therefore RAND application should be limited to cN0 or cN+ necks without evident ECS on preoperative examination. Most of the advantages of RAND result from the incision being remotely placed. Considering the area of dissection, it is not more invasive than the traditional transcervical ND. The robotic system merely helps the surgeon to dissect the lymphatic tissue where access would be troublesome. Despite all these advantages of RAND, improving the cosmetic result is a secondary issue in ND and should never compromise oncologic safety. A considerable portion of RAND is performed under gross vision (levels IIa, IIb, III, and Va). In our experience, the numbers of lymph nodes retrieved for each type of RAND were comparable with those for its conventional counterpart (data not shown).

Moreover, the procedure should be conducted with minimal complications or morbidities. Therefore, RAND should be conducted after sufficient acquisition of surgical anatomy and experience of CND. Because the robotic procedure is conducted in a lateral to medial direction, experiencing CND in the same manner may be helpful to

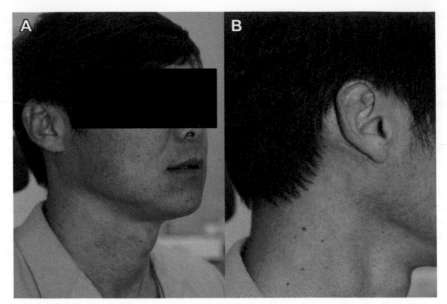

Fig. 18. After surgery. (*A*) Robot-assisted SND level I to III for oral tongue cancer. (*B*) Robot-assisted MRND for tonsillar cancer. Postoperative scar is hidden by the auricle and hair without any significant lymphedema or fibrotic change of the dissected area.

shorten the learning curve and the operation times. Long-term results for oncologic safety and functional outcomes are required to establish the validity of RAND. In addition, a clear and important contraindication to RAND using the RA or MFL incision is the N3 neck and/or the presence of ECS.[31]

REFERENCES

1. Rumsey N, Clarke A, White P. Exploring the psychosocial concerns of outpatients with disfiguring conditions. J Wound Care 2003;12:247.
2. Koh YW, Park JH, Kim JW, et al. Clipless and sutureless endoscopic thyroidectomy using only the Harmonic scalpel. Surg Endosc 2010;24:1117.
3. Kim HS, Chung SM, Pae SY, et al. Endoscope assisted submandibular sialadenectomy: The face-lift approach. Eur Arch Otorhinolaryngol 2011;268:619.
4. Song CM, Jung YH, Sung MW, et al. Endoscopic resection of the submandibular gland via a hairline incision: a new surgical approach. Laryngoscope 2010;120:970.
5. Chen WL, Fang SL. Removal of second branchial cleft cysts using a retroauricular approach. Head Neck 2009;31:695.
6. Roh JL. Retroauricular hairline incision for removal of upper neck masses. Laryngoscope 2005;115:216.
7. Roh JL. Removal of the submandibular gland by a retroauricular approach. Arch Otolaryngol Head Neck Surg 2006;132:783.
8. Lee HS, Lee D, Koo YC, et al. Endoscopic resection of upper neck masses via retroauricular approach is feasible with excellent cosmetic outcomes. J Oral Maxillofac Surg 2013;71(3):520–7.
9. Koh YW, Park JH, Kim JW, et al. Endoscopic hemithyroidectomy with prophylactic ipsilateral central neck dissection via an unilateral axillo-breast approach without

gas insufflation for unilateral micropapillary thyroid carcinoma: preliminary report. Surg Endosc 2010;24(1):188–97.

10. Koh YW, Kim JW, Lee SW, et al. Endoscopic thyroidectomy via a unilateral axillo-breast approach without gas insufflation for unilateral benign thyroid lesions. Surg Endosc 2009;23(9):2053–60.

11. Lee HS, Park do Y, Hwang CS, et al. Feasibility of robot-assisted submandibular gland resection via retroauricular approach: preliminary results. Laryngoscope 2013;123(2):369–73.

12. Lee HS, Kim D, Lee SY, et al. Robot-assisted versus endoscopic submandibular gland resection via retroauricular approach: a prospective nonrandomized study. Br J Oral Maxillofac Surg 2014;52(2):179–84.

13. Kim CH, Byeon HK, Shin YS, et al. Robot-assisted Sistrunk's operation via a retro-auricular approach for thyroglossal duct cyst. Head Neck 2013;36(3):456–8.

14. Weinstein GS, O'Malley BW Jr, Snyder W, et al. Transoral robotic surgery: radical tonsillectomy. Arch Otolaryngol Head Neck Surg 2007;133(12):1220–6.

15. Moore EJ, Olsen KD, Martin EJ. Concurrent neck dissection and transoral robotic surgery. Laryngoscope 2011;121(3):541–4.

16. Weinstein GS, Quon H, O'Malley BW Jr, et al. Selective neck dissection and de-intensified postoperative radiation and chemotherapy for oropharyngeal cancer: a subset analysis of the University of Pennsylvania transoral robotic surgery trial. Laryngoscope 2010;120(9):1749–55.

17. Moore EJ, Henstrom DK, Olsen KD, et al. Transoral resection of tonsillar squamous cell carcinoma. Laryngoscope 2009;119(3):508–15.

18. Moore EJ, Olsen KD, Kasperbauer JL. Transoral robotic surgery for oropharyngeal squamous cell carcinoma: a prospective study of feasibility and functional outcomes. Laryngoscope 2009;119(11):2156–64.

19. Genden EM, Desai S, Sung CK. Transoral robotic surgery for the management of head and neck cancer: a preliminary experience. Head Neck 2009;31(3):283–9.

20. Shin YS, Choi EC, Kim CH, et al. Robot-assisted selective neck dissection combined with facelift parotidectomy in parotid cancer. Head Neck 2014;36(4):592–5.

21. Byeon HK, Holsinger FC, Koh YW, et al. Endoscopic supraomohyoid neck dissection via a retroauricular or modified facelift approach: preliminary results. Head Neck 2014;36(3):425–30.

22. Kim CH, Koh YW, Kim D, et al. Robotic-assisted neck dissection in submandibular gland cancer: preliminary report. J Oral Maxillofac Surg 2013;71(8):1450–7.

23. Park YM, Holsinger FC, Kim WS, et al. Robot-assisted selective neck dissection of levels II to V via a modified facelift or retroauricular approach. Otolaryngol Head Neck Surg 2013;148(5):778–85.

24. Kim CH, Chang JW, Choi EC, et al. Robotically assisted selective neck dissection in parotid gland cancer: preliminary report. Laryngoscope 2013;123(3):646–50.

25. Park YM, Lee WJ, Yun IS, et al. Free flap reconstruction after robot-assisted neck dissection via a modified face-lift or retroauricular approach. Ann Surg Oncol 2013;20(3):891–8.

26. Byeon HK, Ban MJ, Lee JM, et al. Robot-assisted Sistrunk's operation, total thyroidectomy, and neck dissection via a transaxillary and retroauricular (TARA) approach in papillary carcinoma arising in thyroglossal duct cyst and thyroid gland. Ann Surg Oncol 2012;19(13):4259–61.

27. Lee HS, Kim WS, Hong HJ, et al. Robot-assisted supraomohyoid neck dissection via a modified face-lift or retroauricular approach in early-stage cN0 squamous

cell carcinoma of the oral cavity: a comparative study with conventional technique. Ann Surg Oncol 2012;19(12):3871–8.

28. Shin YS, Hong HJ, Koh YW, et al. Gasless transaxillary robot-assisted neck dissection: a preclinical feasibility study in four cadavers. Yonsei Med J 2012; 53(1):193–7.

29. Koh YW, Chung WY, Hong HJ, et al. Robot-assisted selective neck dissection via modified face-lift approach for early oral tongue cancer: a video demonstration. Ann Surg Oncol 2012;19(4):1334–5.

30. Kim WS, Lee HS, Kang SM, et al. Feasibility of robot-assisted neck dissections via a transaxillary and retroauricular ("TARA") approach in head and neck cancer: preliminary results. Ann Surg Oncol 2012;19(3):1009–17.

31. Kim WS, Byeon HK, Park YM, et al. Therapeutic robot-assisted neck dissection via a retroauricular or modified face lift approach in head and neck cancer: A comparative study with conventional transcervical neck dissection. Head Neck 2013 Dec 24. [Epub ahead of print].

Index

Note: Page numbers of article titles are in **boldface** type.

B

Bleeding, postoperative, following robot-assisted neck dissection, 447

C

Carotid artery, medially displaced, 364
Chyle leakage, in lymphatic/thoracic duct injury, following robot-assisted neck dissection, 447
Computed tomography, preoperative, for transoral robotic surgery, 364
Cranial fossa, anterior, approach to, for robotic surgery, 416–417

D

da Vinci robot, parts of, 407

E

Endoscopy, staging, for transoral robotic surgery of oropharynx, 364

F

Facelift thyroidectomy, robotic. See *Thyroidectomy, robotic facelift.*

H

Hair loss at skin incision, following robot-assisted neck dissection, 448
Hematoma, postoperative, following robot-assisted neck dissection, 447
Human papillomavirus-associated oropharyngeal squamous cell carcinoma, 359
Hypertrophic scar, following robot-assisted neck dissection, 448
Hypopharyngeal lesions, transoral robotic surgery for, patient setup for, 411
    surgical technique for, 411–412
Hypopharynx, transoral robotic surgery of, postoperative management of, 412

I

Infratemporal fossa, approach to, for robotic surgery, 419

K

Keloid formation, following robot-assisted neck dissection, 448

L

Laryngectomy, supraglottic, for transoral robotic surgery, in laryngeal cancer, 383–385
    total, for transoral robotic surgery, in laryngeal cancer, 385–388

Otolaryngol Clin N Am 47 (2014) 455–459
http://dx.doi.org/10.1016/S0030-6665(14)00045-0
oto.theclinics.com
0030-6665/14/$ – see front matter © 2014 Elsevier Inc. All rights reserved.

Printed and bound by CPI Group (UK) Ltd, Croydon, CR0 4YY

03/10/2024

01040496-0014